Rural Tranquillity to National Crisis:

A Farm Vet's Story

Copyright © David Harwood 2015

Published by 5m Publishing
Benchmark House
8 Smithy Wood Drive
Sheffield
S35 1QN
United Kingdom

www.5mpublishing.com
books@5mpublishing.com

Cover images by Rachael Meyer of SiRA Studio. http://sirastudio.com

ISBN: 978-1-910455-01-2
A CIP catalogue record for this book is available from the British Library.

Printed and bound in the UK

Rural Tranquillity to National Crisis:

A Farm Vet's Story

David Harwood

Contents

	Foreword	vii
	Introduction	ix
	Dedication	xi
	Acknowledgements	xi
1	1950: Baby Boom Year in a Quiet Worcestershire Village	1
2	Market Gardening in the Vale of Evesham	7
3	My Early Fascination with Animal Husbandry	13
4	Pigs, Horses, Goats and Sheep – a Grammar School Education!	21
5	How Veterinary College Life has Changed!	29
6	Do I Really Need to Know All This?	41
7	The Pressure Mounts – Final Exams Approach	51
8	A Vet at Last – but Stress Levels Rise Again!	67
9	It's a Farm Vet for Me – Devon Beckons	89
10	Over the Border to Dorset	103
11	A 'Man from the Ministry', and Back to My Studies!	115
12	Veterinary Detective Work on the Front Line	125
13	Mad Cows and an Englishman	149
14	A National Crisis Unfolds – I Head Out onto the Front Line	161
15	Less Disinfectant – and a Move to the Control Teams	177
16	You've Got to be Kidding!	189
17	Some Final Thoughts	197

Foreword

Almost exactly six years before I read this book I walked nervously into a rather daunting room at the headquarters of the British Veterinary Association. It was my first meeting as a trustee of the Animal Welfare Foundation (AWF) and I had no idea what to expect. What I didn't expect at all was to fall in love. But that's exactly what happened.

David Harwood joined the AWF on the same day as me and I've been smitten ever since. Don't get too excited; there is no infidelity worthy of a tabloid headline about to be announced, simply the fact that he is one of those people you instantly feel like you've known for your whole life but can't quite remember why. Luckily for those unfortunate souls among you who will never get the opportunity to meet him, you can drink in the warmth of this wonderful man through the words of his story.

There have been so many books written about the lives of those of us who ended up with the not-so-proverbial 'hand up a cow's arse' that you could ask yourself why you should read another. There are two answers to that question. The first is that being a vet, any vet, is a life so full of extremes – from tragedy to side-splitting, irreverent hilarity – that every vet on the planet would be able to tell you *something* about the madness of owners that you hadn't heard before. And secondly, David has had a life quite different to the vast majority of vets in run-of-the-mill practices.

He mentions one of his bosses, a real role model, who had what he describes as 'a twinkle in his eye'. I think David may be wonderfully unaware that this is just how I think of him. When he told me at one of our charity meetings that he was writing his life story for his family I knew I wanted to read it. The twinkle in his eye whenever he relates anything that has happened or is about to happen draws you in and his mischievous but slightly enigmatic smile leaves you sure you will want to know more.

You will hear about the decades gone by that will evoke strong memories, both good and bad, in all of you. You will hear about those mad, bad animals and their much madder owners – but you will also take a journey into the mysterious shadowy world of... THE MINISTRY. I think it sounded much darker and more Orwellian before the Ministry of Agriculture changed its name to DEFRA but our enigmatic David was there throughout. Like a spy worthy of that twinkle he had to have the manuscript approved from on high because of the secrets he *could* have revealed. We may have to wait for the whistle-blowing but the stories he can tell from those days are what makes this book stand apart from the others. There are very few vets who were dealing with disease outbreaks and were on the frontline of discovering the new diseases which have shaped the history of our country.

BSE may seem like something from the past but for those of us who were alive when it was discovered it was a very scary thing indeed. 'Mad Cow Disease', as it was called, may have been a godsend to the creators of *Spitting Image* but it certainly conjured up all our demons when we found out that humans could catch it. In the book David unravels BSE and Foot-and-Mouth Disease along with many other weird and not-so-wonderful diseases which have changed thousands of lives forever.

Of course, outside of the clinical setting of the laboratory the heart-breaking stories of mass destruction that come with all these disease outbreaks are only too real. The obvious affection that David had for the devastated people involved is a great testament not only to him but to vets the world over.

I feel like I want to tell you all the gems you are about to hear but I must stop myself. We'll have to get together for a drink and a natter to do that once you've read it too. *Rural Tranquillity* not only tells the tale of this modest, endearing man but is an eye-widening reminder of what hasn't changed about being a vet contrasted starkly with what has. Suffice to say that I'm pleased to know that crashing the practice car repeatedly is, as I long hoped, not something that is unique to me!

As for you, get yourself a cup of tea or a glass of wine, unplug your phone, put a Do Not Disturb sign on your forehead and prepare yourself to fall in love all over again.

Emma Milne

Introduction

When my mother in her 84th year paid a visit to the school in the village where she lived, an archive copy of the register displayed her name and that of my late father. They were both born in the village of Church Lench in Worcestershire and stayed there for the remainder of their lives. Many of their childhood friends had also stayed in the same village.

I have been part of the first generation of which a high proportion have migrated from their childhood homes to pursue their careers and aspirations as university places and employment opportunities became more widely available further afield. Social media websites such as Friends Reunited and Facebook have confirmed just how widely distributed my childhood friends are today.

I was born in 1950 at a time when the British way of life was still recovering after the end of the Second World War. A trip to my local supermarket today, with its vast array of food products from around the world, makes it difficult for me to comprehend that food rationing in post-war Britain did not end until I was four years old.

My idyllic upbringing in this quiet and isolated Worcestershire village, walking alongside the horses with my grandfather as they ploughed the fields and picking fruit throughout the summer, is a far cry from village life today. Church Lench is now within easy commuter distance of Birmingham and, as a result, has attracted a diverse range of families from all over the country. My mother and her childhood friends are now among a small minority of people who have lived there all their lives, yet due to the local interest in village history, they are frequently asked to tell the stories of the past that I remember so well.

My grandfather, Albert Allen, was in awe of the local vet from Evesham, who made regular visits to the village farm where my grandfather worked as a stockman. I spent many happy days 'helping' my grandfather and gradually began to realise that I loved farm work and farm animals. Indeed, by the time I was nine, I could only imagine becoming a vet as a future career. Sadly, my grandfather died in my early teens, but my ambition to become a vet never left me. In 1969, I entered the Royal Veterinary College, University of London, as the first member of my family to go to university. Five years later I achieved my lifelong ambition of qualifying as a veterinary surgeon.

This autobiography takes the reader on a journey from my early, very rural life in post-war Britain, through the trials and tribulations of getting into veterinary school in London, an environment far removed from that of my village. It compares and contrasts the university course and student life in the computer-free 1970s with that of the modern veterinary degree and its changing student base. The journey continues into my life as a veterinary surgeon, with probably more changes seen by my profession during the span of my career than at any equivalent timespan before, particularly as the technological era evolved.

My early time as a vet was spent in mixed practice, but I gradually specialised in farm work during my time in Devon in the 1970s and in Dorset during the late 1970s and early 1980s, before a career change diverted me to work as a veterinary investigation officer in the government's State Veterinary Service (SVS).

As a government vet for most of my career, I experienced the arrival of bovine spongiform encephalopathy (BSE) and the impact it had on British farming. I spent nearly a year dealing with the 2001 foot-and-mouth disease (FMD) epidemic, followed by further involvement during the 2007 outbreak.

The majority of my time working for the government was, however, spent investigating farm animal diseases on an individual and flock/herd basis in an attempt to ensure that UK livestock remained fit, healthy and profitable, and that farm animal welfare did not suffer as a result. This routine work also enabled the SVS to identify the unusual – what we referred to as new and emerging diseases – indeed the recognition of BSE was a prime example of this. Another part of our remit was to ensure consumer safety and confidence in the milk and meat originating from UK livestock units.

The characters I have met and the individual animal cases I remember are all firmly imprinted on my mind – and are memories desperate to be shared! Above all, however, it is the immense change that has occurred in both the veterinary and the wider world that has influenced my decision to write this book.

Dedication

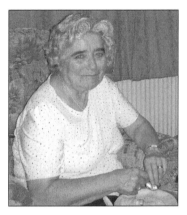

To my mother Joyce Taylor (Harwood) who was my original inspiration to sit down and look back at my life. Sadly as the final editing process was being completed she died aged 86 on December 2nd 2014 after a long battle with Non-Hodgkin Lymphoma – which as with everything else in her long life she faced with incredible bravery and positivity.

To my sister Carol and my step-father Pat who have given her such loving support during this cruel illness.

To my father Malcolm Harwood who died so young at only 54.

Last and by no means least to my wife Gerry, my daughters Maddy and Jess and my stepdaughters Nicola and Kimberley for always being there for me.

Acknowledgements

I have already named many in the text who have inspired me along the way. The Royal Veterinary College year of 1974 and the staff who taught us deserve a special mention, as do my fellow colleagues and friends who worked with me in MAFF / Defra in the Veterinary Investigation Service (as it was originally known – and still referred to despite its many name changes).

Any photo attributed incorrectly to the author is regretted.

Chapter 1

1950: Baby Boom Year in a Quiet Worcestershire Village

I came into the world on 17 January 1950, the first-born son of Joyce and Malcolm Harwood, both only 22 years old and married in 1948 in the aftermath of the Second World War. My parents were born and grew up in the Worcestershire village of Church Lench, in the Vale of Evesham – at that time a thriving and vibrant market gardening area.

Although I grew up the son of a market gardener, it was my grandfather, the stockman on a local small mixed farm, and the farm vet Geoffrey Bowler who ignited my interest in becoming a vet. It was an ambition I carried with me from the age of nine until I eventually entered the Royal Veterinary College in 1969, qualifying as a vet five years later.

Almost 40 years on, I can reflect that I have experienced an unprecedented number of changes in both my personal and veterinary life in that time. Along the way I have met some fascinating characters, many of whom will feature in this book. Some were inspirational, some were amusing and some were frustrating – but all have played their part.

The UK post-war baby boom was mirrored in Church Lench and I was the first of a number of babies born during 1950. My sister Carol was born almost exactly five years later, on 3 January 1955.

My father was a major fan of cricket and my initials DG (David Graham) were given to me in honour of his then cricketing idol Don Bradman (or DG Bradman as the scorecard displayed his name). I still have an old notebook in which my father recorded the scorecards for test matches and those of his beloved Worcestershire County Cricket Club, all meticulously written in his unmistakable handwriting.

Church Lench is 5½ miles north of Evesham and 13 miles east of Stratford -upon-Avon. Today, it is a vibrant and expanding village with a population of around 600, modern transport networks making it within easy commuting distance of some of the major towns and cities in the Midlands. The name Lench is shared by five villages and comes from an Anglo-Saxon word 'hlinc', meaning 'rising ground or hill'. In descending order of size, they are Church Lench, Rous Lench, Atch Lench, Sheriffs Lench and Ab Lench. Church Lench itself has been in existence for more than a thousand years and is mentioned in the Domesday Book. The settlements of that time belonged to the Great Abbey of Evesham, and All Saints Church in the village can trace its origins back to Saxon and Norman times.

Church Lench had a population of between 350 and 400 in the 1950s and agriculture, in particular market gardening, was the main activity. My father and his father were both market gardeners and we had around six acres, mainly growing plums, with open ground for strawberries and other soft fruit, and brassicas, such as sprouts. We also had around 200 laying hens that spent the winter in two deep litter houses and the summertime keeping the grass down under the fruit trees. One of my early jobs was to shut all the hens in each night to protect them from foxes, always after dark. I can admit now that it was a bit scary at times. In my mind I was never alone – there was always something watching me!

We first lived at Hilltop, a rented black and white timbered cottage across the road from the church. It adjoined Church Farm, a dairy farm run by Wilf Major, who was one of the village's real characters. Across the drive was the village shop, a Co-op, and at that time one of the main focuses of village life. It was a regular meeting place for my mother and her friends.

My Aunty Kath kept the village post office, which was literally in the hallway of her house down the road from the shop. Every Friday, a travelling hardware van owned by Wards stopped in the village. It carried all the other essentials including paraffin, which had a lingering smell I can remember vividly.

Although we had electricity at the time, many more rural locations such as my grandfather's farm did not. We had no mains water – that didn't arrive for several years – and we all relied on the communal water pump in the backyard.

While we were living at Hilltop, my parents decided to take the big step of buying a television set, which few people owned at the time. Although the main excuse was to watch the Queen's coronation on 2 June 1953, I later realised that it was the televised cricket that was being increasingly broadcast that also played a part! Even though I was only three, I can remember our neighbours sitting in our living room watching the small black and white screen contained in a huge wooden box standing in the corner of the room. How different are our giant flatscreen TVs of today. As the television needed an aerial to be positioned on the roof or chimney, our landlord, who was apparently very wary of this new technology, worried that such an addition might have an adverse effect on the chimney structure so he very cleverly put up the rent 'just in case your aerial damages my roof'.

It was the radio, however, that I remember listening to, with programmes such as *Uncle Mac's Children's Hour* and *Children's Favourites*. Songs that I grew up listening to included *Sparky's Magic Piano*, *Nellie the Elephant*, *How Much is that Doggie in the Window*, *You're a Pink Toothbrush* and *I Taut I Taw a Puddy Tat*. The radio was always on in the background as I grew up and our traditional Sunday lunch would never be Sunday lunch without *Two Way Family Favourites* on in the background. This was a very popular record request programme designed to link families at home in the UK with British Forces Posted Overseas (BFPO). Its forerunner was aired during the Second World War and titled *Forces Favourites*. Soldiers and their families at home could request a favourite record, along with a personal dedication. At the end of the war, the show was renamed *Family Favourites* and broadcast on the Light Programme. The original format was expanded in 1960 to a longer 90-minute Sunday show, with two announcers linked by telephone. One presenter was based in London, the other in a BFPO station in Canada, West Germany, Singapore, Hong Kong or Australia. The two presenters I remember from that time were Jean Metcalfe and Cliff Michelmore.

Children's television in the 1950s was a developing medium and I was lucky enough to be able to sit and watch many of those early programmes. The afternoon children's slot was broadcast as *Watch with Mother* and had a different short slot each day. Monday was *Picture Book*, which gave ideas for things to make and do. On Tuesday, it was *Andy Pandy*, followed on Wednesday by *The Flowerpot Men*, who, to me as a young boy, seemed quite believable, but to an adult somewhat strange. With their 'flibadobs' and 'flobadobs' as their only way of talking, the Flowerpot Men Bill and Ben lived in two giant flowerpots at the bottom of the garden, behind the potting shed. Keeping a lookout for them was Little Weed, who warned them if anyone approached so they could hide! On Thursday, it was the turn of *Rag, Tag and Bobtail*, which concerned the adventures of a hedgehog, a mouse and a rabbit. The Friday slot was occupied by the *The Woodentops*, in which Daddy Woodentop was always busy doing 'men's work' and Mummy Woodentop was busy in the kitchen assisted by Mrs Scrubbit. In addition to the Woodentop children, the family also had Buttercup the Cow and a rascal of a hound called Spotty Dog, who was referred to as 'the biggest spotty dog you ever did see'.

Another popular programme of my childhood was *The Sooty Show*, the glove puppet creation of Harry Corbett. Many years later, around 1980, when I was a member of Blandford Forum Round Table, I appeared on stage dressed as a chicken doing *The Birdie Song* with Sooty and Sweep, ably assisted by Harry and his wife, who lived nearby.

In the 1950s and 1960s cowboy programmes were very popular and these included *The Lone Ranger*, *Rawhide* and *Wells Fargo*. I was also an avid fan of *Circus Boy* starring the ten-year-old Micky Dolenz, who would later become a member of the pop group The Monkees.

Today, children have such a vast array of entertainment media at their disposal, from countless satellite channels, DVDs and an endless supply of video games. However, thanks to YouTube, it is also possible to revisit one's childhood television and radio experiences.

I was a naughty and mischievous boy, according to my mother. I even attempted to leave home at the age of four by running down a street, which thankfully was almost empty of traffic. My mother told me many years later that I had told her I was leaving – I have no idea why – and she played along with it, even making me a sandwich to take with me. She told me she closed the door as I left and watched me through the letterbox, knowing full well I would quickly return, which of course I did.

We used to pay regular visits to my mother's parents, both of whom lived around the corner, and to my father's mother (my paternal grandfather died before I was born, my father being the youngest of eight). I was apparently at my worst when visiting Granny Harwood, often with my cousin Anne, who by contrast, and much to my mother's frustration, was angelic compared to me and only made my behaviour look worse. Apparently, my chief misdemeanour was to hide under the dining table, pulling off the cloth and its contents and then liberally spreading the dust that had accumulated on the struts of the table to watch it fall to the ground. Anne, of course, sat quietly watching.

One particular event has stuck in my mind from my early years and it probably had quite a profound influence on me. My father was in hospital at the time and we had a serious chimney fire. My mother quite understandably panicked and we had to call the fire brigade. From that day on, I was extremely wary of fire and I would not strike a match for many years. On a more positive note, it is maybe one of the reasons I have never tried smoking, even though both of my parents smoked when I was young.

After Granny Harwood died, my parents decided to buy her house and six acres of land across the road. Thus started a new chapter in my life, when I would have been around six years old. As the move was less than half a mile away and as finances were always tight, my father asked a friend who owned a lorry to help us move.

I can quite clearly remember the event, as I was allowed to sit on the lorry with our belongings. My most vivid and light-hearted memory, however, was also the reason my mother tried to forget the whole incident. In order not to attract too much attention so 'folks wouldn't see our belongings', the move took place at dusk. However, the smooth, almost covert, event was quickly revealed by one of the helpers on the back of the lorry because he played my mother's piano all the way from the old house to the new one!

The Poplars, as our new house was called, was a detached house with four bedrooms and our own water pump. We were to live there for the next ten years and it was in this home that I suppose everything began for me. While I lived there I passed the 11-plus, started at Prince Henry's Grammar School in Evesham and did my O-levels.

It was also in this house that I eventually learned the truth about Father Christmas when he, or in this case she, woke me up, as my mother banged the door frame with my main gift, a guitar, as she came into the room. I did not tell her I knew the secret until much later.

I had already started at the village primary school when we moved, the same one my parents had attended. There were two classes, called with great imagination 'little class' and 'big class', with two teachers, Mr Walker and Miss Harris the headmistress. My primary school life was fairly uneventful, although I do regret the fact (my fault not theirs) that, although I left with a sound all round primary education, I also left with dreadful handwriting that I retain to this day. I was constantly criticised for this throughout both my primary and secondary schooling, but Nan (my mother's mother) used to defend me by saying my brain was working so fast, my hand simply couldn't keep up. Thanks Nan, I have been using that same excuse now for years.

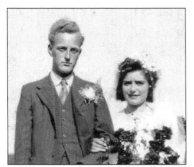

My mother and father Joyce and Malcolm on their wedding day.

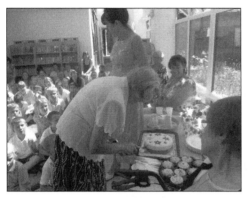

My mother at 85 opening a new classroom in Church Lench primary school where both my parents and my sister and I all attended.

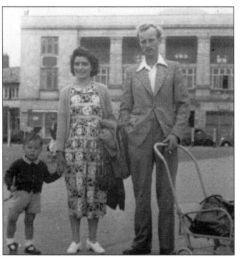

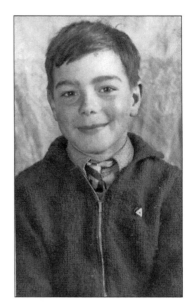

Primary school photograph.

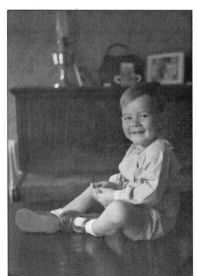

Me aged around 4.

Family day out wth my parents.

Chapter 2
Market Gardening in the Vale of Evesham

When we moved to The Poplars, we took over the land across the road, which was mainly a plum orchard. Several years later we also took over an apple orchard and some derelict land we then cleared and replanted with more fruit trees. Market gardening was the main source of our family income for the next few years and was also a source of extra pocket money for me.

It may seem obvious, but market gardening is exactly what it sounds like – the skill of cultivating the land you have to produce crops you can sell at market. I still have my father's favourite hand tool, a wooden handled, four-tined and very pointed rake, used to great effect in breaking down the soil, raking it over, and hoeing between plants and rows. I still refer to it as a scratter, the name my father always used. You never see them sold anywhere now, probably due yet again to health and safety concerns that the user may injure themselves or someone around them with the sharp points. My father had a particular ability to sow and plant with incredibly consistent success. He would give me six young sprout plants for my garden in later years and, if I were lucky, four would grow to full size. He would plant 2,000, and 1,998 would grow to be healthy and productive plants.

The vagaries of the market at this time could rapidly turn against him. I remember two marketing disasters very clearly and the frustration and disappointment my father must have felt. We had an excellent crop of runner beans one year, but so did everyone else. Our baskets remained unsold in the Evesham fruit and veg wholesale auction market and were subsequently dumped. The cost to us was the market commission. Similarly, we planted, weeded, pulled, washed and tied spring onions. One week they sold well, in other weeks of glut they did not and yet again they were dumped, leaving us with another commission bill.

It was a real family business and we all played our part. I remember sitting on boxes surrounded by heaps of spring onions my father had pulled. My mother, father and sister all selected the right number of onions for the bunch size (not too big or too small) and placed an elastic band around the bundle. They then 'tagged' them – effectively pulling off any yellowing leaves – then 'topped' them by breaking off the leaves at one end to leave a straight and uniform line. The onions were then washed and packed in boxes ready to go to market where, fingers crossed, they would sell. I earned the sum of one halfpenny per bunch. As all the fruit picking and other tasks were effectively 'piece work', I rapidly picked up speed, keeping a constant note in my head of what I had earned.

One particularly enjoyable task was redcurrant picking, and we had quite a few bushes to pick. This was a 'sitting down on a stool task', delicately picking off the strings of berries so as not to damage them. Strawberry picking was less enjoyable and was back-breaking work, but nevertheless both supplemented my pocket money.

The Vale of Evesham was always known for its plum crop, particularly the local dessert variety called yellow egg or Pershore egg. This type probably represented around three-quarters of our total crop. We also grew Victoria, purple egg, czars and damsons.

During the 1960s, there were many smallholdings growing plums in the village, including strips of land either side of us. Every year when it was considered the white plum blossom would be at its best, there was a designated Blossom Sunday, with the blue RAC signs marking a circular route around the Vale of Evesham, including through Church Lench. The usually quiet village streets were then host to a steady stream of cars and even coaches, many of which had travelled from neighbouring towns and cities such as Birmingham to view the blossom.

A popular pastime on these days was collecting car numbers – literally writing the registration numbers of cars passing through the village into a notebook. Looking back on this, it does show how we could make our own entertainment (and we did have competitions between my friends to see who could collect the most), without the need for the elaborate computer and other games that entertain children today. The highlight of each Blossom Sunday, however, was the long procession of cars that were forced to follow Wilf Major's cows as he slowly drove them from their fields along the village road to his farm next to the church for milking. Cars were going so slowly that drivers often shouted out their registration numbers to us as they drove past – it really was a popular pastime! The return journey of the cows against the flow of traffic was also memorable, watching town and city car owners panic as the cows came towards them, often brushing up against the cars as they walked past. The sight of cow muck all over the road was not unusual and, in those days, no one took pride in the grass verge outside their house – it wasn't worth it.

The start of the plum picking season itself was heralded by the local wholesalers delivering the wooden boxes or bushels, which each held around 40 to 50 pounds of plums when level full. Before we filled them with plums, my friends Andrew and Sam used to help me make a den in the centre of the pile of boxes.

Quite by chance, in 2013 – some 40 years since I had last seen these boxes – I spotted some in a fashionable store in Winchester, each painted a different colour and filled with a variety of fashion accessories. They caught my eye partly due to their instantly recognisable shape, but also the words JM Stokes and Frank Idiens were clearly written on the side and visible through their new colours. These were the two main wholesalers in Evesham that supplied our boxes and bought our plums. I wonder if these boxes were ever used by us.

When picking began, yet again it was a family affair with all of us picking into a 'peck' wicker basket either worn around our waist or over our shoulder. When we had filled this we tipped it into the waiting boxes, gently so as not to damage the fruit. When I was young and could reach, I would pick the plums on the lower branches. As I became older and stronger, I was promoted to ladders alongside my father, picking plums at the tops of the trees, many of which were old and getting quite high. I remember thinking it wasn't fair that my sister stuck with the rich and easy pickings at the bottom of the tree, while I was moving my ladder around to reach the plums nearer the top. It certainly made me a faster picker as I wanted to pick more than Carol.

We were told quite firmly by my father not to damage the 'bearers' on the trees. We had to gently pull the plums off and not snatch them as this would break off these delicate shoots. However, my uncle and my father's older brother seemed to ignore this rule and the trees he picked from were strewn with these shoots, much to my father's frustration.

After our plum crop had been picked, I managed to get some work in the late summer and early autumn apple and pear picking on the farm where my grandfather had worked. The livestock side had been gradually phased out and the farm had taken over neighbouring apple and pear orchards, mainly Worcester Pearmain apples and Conference pears. Trees were much shorter and ladder work was minimal, so I could quickly fill many boxes in a working day. This was to become a good source of income in my final years at school and early years at veterinary college. I bought my first car, a red Mini with registration number 605 KOF (known affectionately as 'old kof'), for the princely sum of £150 purely out of the proceeds of my summer and autumn fruit picking.

On the subject of cars, very few people owned them even though the village was very isolated during the 1950s and early 1960s. There was just one bus each day, plus a lunchtime service on a Thursday. I used to travel pillion on my father's

BSA motorbike, neither of us wearing a crash helmet. My father then decided to learn to drive, eventually passing his test, and we then bought our first four-wheeled vehicle. It was an Austin A35 green van, registration 729 DFK, with its characteristic orange indicator 'wings' that shot up at right angles when you intended to turn left or right.

This purchase also heralded the start of another phase in our family life, that of retail greengrocer. Having suffered the disappointments of growing our crops only to see them fail to sell and be dumped and, at the other end of the spectrum, witnessing what the housewife paid for produce she bought each week, we decided to cut out the middle man. This small van was used by my parents to develop a mobile greengrocery service in Bromsgrove. This proved to be very successful and resulted in the purchase of increasingly larger vans with shelving that shoppers could walk inside.

We used to visit the wholesalers at Evesham (mainly Frank Sharp), to supplement our own produce with those commodities we could not grow, such as bananas and oranges. I started going along on Saturdays to help run the errands between the van and front doors, taking orders and then ferrying the fruit and vegetables back. We had mainly regular customers, so the van followed the same route each time. Some of these customers we knew by name, others we did not. I developed a real affection for one woman who gave us an order each week, but I never got to know her name. Throughout my time helping out she was always referred to as 'the lady with the bucket', simply because she used to give me a white enamelled bucket to carry items back to the house.

A few years later, we took over a store in Briar Close in Evesham, a typical corner shop selling a variety of items from fresh vegetables and sweets to bags of coal and candles. My mother loved the shop, and pretty well ran it, while my father continued with the mobile greengrocery. My father occasionally worked in the shop, and although he seemed to enjoy his role selling to adult customers, he used to get quite frustrated with the young children who were regular visitors with or without their parents. Being a corner shop, it had a sweet counter, and many of the sweets were on display on shelves in a glass-fronted display case at 'child level'. As they made their choices, my dad had to get down on his knees to pick out their favourite ½ pence chews, lollipops or sherbet. His wicked sense of humour (or in this case, veiled sarcasm) was often evident when he was presented with an indecisive child who made him make several visits on bended knee; he would tell them how 'pleased' he was that they kept him so fit!

I fondly watch old episodes of *Open All Hours*, the BBC sitcom starring Ronnie Barker as Arkwright and David Jason as his long-suffering assistant Granville, and think back to the days when we had a shop which bore more than a striking resemblance to the one featured. We had our share of characters that you could easily slot into the programme, including my father as Evesham's own Arkwright!

One regular task I helped my father with, however, has preyed on my mind ever since. This was the winter tar oil spraying of the fruit trees, designed to control pests and diseases that could damage the trees and their crops. My jobs were to mix the neat tar oil and water to the correct concentration, to ensure that the extractor pipe remained below the fluid level at all times, and to then transfer the pipe to the next barrel. My father did all the spraying himself wearing an old mac and hat, with his customary cigarette in his mouth. Health and safety laws have banned the use of this material since 2004 and, even before the ban, there was strict advice on how to handle such material safely. But this was not so in the 1960s and 1970s. My father's cigarette was yellow (as was his face) from the droplets of spray that covered him. I am as certain as I can be that the particularly invasive lung carcinoma that developed when he was aged just 52, and from which he eventually died at the cruelly young age of 54, was in part due to inhaling not only cigarette smoke, but the toxic breakdown products of the tar oil itself. He was to live for only one year and two days in the life of my eldest daughter, Maddy, and never met Jessica, my youngest daughter. How I wish he had been around for many more years. I still miss him.

How Evesham has changed today. The orchards that once surrounded the village on every side have almost all been destroyed and the hedgerows removed. In their place are wide open fields with the major arable crop now oilseed rape – its vivid yellow flowers looking strangely out of place in the village I knew so well and grew up in.

Chapter 3
My Early Fascination with Animal Husbandry

It was my grandfather and his visiting veterinary surgeon who I feel played the greatest role in my later career choice. That said, I was surrounded by many other memorable pet and livestock influences in my early years.

We never owned a dog as my father simply did not like them. We did, however, adopt a family of semi-wild cats when we took over The Poplars and its land. Their role was to keep down the numbers of rats and mice, which they did particularly well. None of them was ever neutered, so their numbers were always potentially increasing. One cat in particular, who for some unknown reason we all referred to as Granny Cat, was a breeder extraordinaire! I have no idea how many litters of kittens she produced, but she developed the ability to suddenly turn up with three new kittens, which she presented to us like a magician pulling a rabbit from a hat. She was undoubtedly almost single-handedly responsible for cat numbers escalating to a situation where we had to do something to control them. Bearing in mind they were semi-wild, we coaxed them into a shed to feed and then my father and I put our lives at risk by going in with them to catch the ones we wanted to have put down. We finished up with cats seemingly flying around the shed along the roof and walls until, both of us covered in scratches and bites, we had them boxed up. These unlucky ones were then taken to the vet in Evesham to be put to sleep.

We decided that we did need to keep some cats back, including Granny, who quickly became pregnant again. When she had obviously had her kittens somewhere, I was given the task to follow her to find out where they were. This task quickly took on a John Le Carré approach, with me the spy and Granny my target. She often outsmarted me by quickly doubling back on herself, or darting through thick hedges she seemed to know I couldn't follow her through. She would often simply stop, sit and wash herself, and I remember standing idly by pretending to do something else until she thought I'd lost interest, before she set off again. I did, however, begin to find the litters she'd hidden, and we began to control numbers by putting to sleep these new-born kittens. Although I hate to admit it, this was by drowning, a procedure I could not now condone.

As with most children, there comes a time when you want a pet of your own. In my case the choice was easy, we had semi-wild cats that were gradually becoming less wild as I spent more time with them. We let Granny keep one of her next litter and this became my first real pet. Although Granny wasn't keen on me muscling in on the rearing of her kitten, I began to spend more time with her, whom I named Mitzi. She became the first cat we had spayed when she was old enough and Mitzi soon became used to being a pampered pet, spending more and more time in the house with us.

Unfortunately, although the semi-wild cats all lived in the sheds on our land on one side of the road, we lived in The Poplars on the other side of the road. Mitzi, of course, used to go back and forth across the road and I suppose it was inevitable that, despite there being so few cars on the road, her luck would eventually run out. She was hit by a car while crossing, but survived and we found her on the side of the road, a pitiful sight and obviously in pain. This was my first real hands-on veterinary problem. We took her to the vet in Evesham and he diagnosed a fractured pelvis. There appeared to be no other internal complications and no other musculoskeletal injuries and we were told that with confinement in a box and some tender loving care, she should make a recovery.

It was heartbreaking watching Mitzi move from one position to another and the pain from that shattered pelvis was obvious. Cats often react to pain by spitting and swearing and she was no exception. There were no effective painkillers for cats in those days, but she did make a slow, but quite remarkable recovery. Mitzi did, however, finish up with an unusual gait, walking quite stiff legged with a peculiar 'swaying' movement when viewed from behind. In retrospect, it was very similar to the way the elderly deaf waitress played by Julie Walters moved around in the famous *Two Soups* sketch written by Victoria Wood.

I was also given a pet rabbit called Flopsy. He was a Belgian hare/Flemish Giant cross-breed male, and he was a big rabbit. My father helped make a big hutch for him and I quickly got into the daily routine of collecting dandelions and other plants when in season, and feeding him dry rabbit mix through the winter, with hay to eat and straw bedding. I made a wire run at one stage, and forgot how easily rabbits can dig underneath and escape. He wasn't a brave rabbit, however, and although he ran me ragged trying to catch him, he never moved more than 20 ft from his hutch. I got a female rabbit and began breeding them, not that they needed much encouragement. I began reading up on rabbit keeping, learning the importance of putting the female into the male's hutch, and eventually I had around 15 to 20 rabbits.

One word of warning to rabbit owners – beware of feeding them beetroot! Bearing in mind that I lived on a market gardening smallholding, there was always waste material to feed to my rabbits, and one day it was beetroot. I arrived the next day to what looked like a bloodbath. It was a frosty morning but all I could see was red staining all around the hutches, and actually dripping from the back of one of them. This was a very early diagnostic lesson that not all is what it seems as this wasn't blood, merely the red urine discolouration linked to the beetroot pigment.

My father kept a number of laying hens, so it was only natural I suppose that I should follow suit. But, wanting to be different, I kept bantams. I had a small shed and run, and around six bantams all hatched from fertile eggs I had been given and placed under a broody hen. I tried selling the bantam eggs to my mother or any other family member but with minimal success.

We kept our laying hens partly as a source of additional income from the eggs, but also to keep the grass and weeds down under the fruit trees in the summer. I learned a lot about basic poultry keeping and handling from my father that proved invaluable to me when I started training to be a vet. I learned practical things, such as catching and handling, that I was never taught on the veterinary course itself, and that I've never forgotten.

I've already described my trips down to shut all the birds in at night to keep them safe from the fox. This was always a real battle with the pullets (young pre-laying birds), that preferred to roost in the trees. Foxes have this ability to 'mesmerise' a roosting bird from its perch, so they were not safe. Armed with long poles, we used to literally poke them out of the trees and round them up into the pop-holes of the chicken sheds and this could be a lengthy process, particularly on a cold wet evening. My other roles were feeding and egg collecting, together with egg washing, grading (for size) and storing them on trays in wooden boxes to be collected by the Egg Marketing Board.

The board at that time was an agricultural marketing organisation set up by the Government in December 1956 to stabilise the market for eggs due to a widespread collapse in sales. The board purchased all the eggs produced in the UK, graded them to a national standard, and then marketed them to shops. Each eggshell was stamped with a small lion logo as a mark of quality that would be seen by the customer. We were paid accordingly and docked money for cracked, dirty or misshapen eggs. There were a number of memorable adverts run by the board at that time, with slogans such as 'Go to work on an egg', introduced in 1957, and eventually turned into a series of television advertisements starring

Tony Hancock and featuring Patricia Hayes and Pat Coombs that ran for six years from 1965 to 1971. The board closed down in 1971 and the lion mark was dropped.

During the winter we caught and moved all the birds into two deep litter houses. Frozen water pipes were a constant problem as any interruption in supply was quickly reflected by a dramatic drop in egg production. We manipulated the daylight hours by timer switches to turn on and off lights to lengthen the day and fool the birds that it was summer not winter. This increased their egg output at a time when they naturally lay far fewer eggs. We were also plagued by rats, particularly in one house. With the red dimmer lights on, I was given an airgun to try to kill the vermin as they moved around the building. We were loath to use poison in case it killed either the birds or our cats.

All these activities were subliminally forming a sound animal husbandry basis to my future veterinary career. I was learning skills along the way that were never formally taught to me, and I suspect may still not be on the syllabus in veterinary schools today.

One of my first real hands-on veterinary experiences, however, followed an escalating mortality problem in some young laying birds. Fowl pest (now referred to as Newcastle disease) was a fairly common, but fortunately sporadic, problem around the country in the 1960s and 1970s and we feared we had it. We contacted the local Ministry of Agriculture office and what followed was my introduction to real veterinary work.

The man from the ministry, who was called Eddie Winkler, arrived and, after donning the formidable ministry clothing of long black waterproof coat and black sou'wester, proceeded to inspect our birds. My father told him I hoped to be a vet one day and Eddie was great. He explained to me what he was looking for (respiratory and nervous signs in the remaining live birds), told me he saw nothing of concern and ruled out fowl pest. He then decided to carry out some post-mortem examinations on top of a feed bin in our shed and invited me to watch. Eddie carefully explained the anatomy, a vital basis to understand pathology, before showing me what he thought was wrong. There were tumour lesions developing in some body organs and we were told that the problem was Marek's disease, a poultry problem we still have today but one that is now effectively controlled in the commercial sector by vaccination.

It was around this time that I first took out *Black's Veterinary Dictionary* from Evesham library and began reading it, looking initially at the signs and symptoms of Marek's disease. I had it on almost permanent loan for the next few years!

I can't remember the exact time, but in the early 1960s we did have fowl pest in the village and a number of small poultry flocks including our own were slaughtered compulsorily to control the disease. We had a huge pit dug on the lower part of our land, into which all the birds were tipped and then buried. We were not allowed to re-stock until the buildings had been cleaned and disinfected and the area declared free of disease. The village smelled of disinfectant, and disinfectant-soaked straw mats were placed at the entrance to our land and at all entry points for vehicles into the village.

This procedure was repeated again in 1967, when the country experienced a devastating outbreak of foot-and-mouth disease (only eclipsed in scale by the 2001 outbreak). We had no livestock that were susceptible but the men from the ministry were all around us in their black protective clothing, setting up road blocks and disinfection sites and carrying out inspections of susceptible livestock. This included all cloven-hoofed animals, such as cattle, sheep, pigs and goats. The disease was confirmed in Worcestershire and sadly Wilf Major's beloved cows were destroyed in the desperate attempts to control the outbreak.

As a veterinary surgeon, I was later to be heavily involved in the mammoth efforts to control and contain the devastating outbreak in 2001 and the smaller localised outbreak in 2007, both potential national crises.

One of our next-door neighbours was known to us as Amy and she had a passion for her goats, which she kept purely as a hobby. I have met so many more 'Amys' over the years and am always impressed with their passion for these fascinating and gentle creatures. I developed a real interest in goat health and welfare during my veterinary career and I am currently an honorary veterinary surgeon to the British Goat Society.

I must have been aged about nine when I first decided I wanted to be a vet when I left school and this desire became more focused and consolidated as I grew into my teens. My passion for farm work, however, which I have focused on throughout most of my career, and my initial inspiration both came from my grandfather and the vet who visited his farm.

My grandfather did not own the farm, he was an employed stockman and looked after a small herd of beef cattle, some breeding sows and fattening pigs, some laying hens and turkeys for the Christmas market.

I spent many days with my grandfather as a young boy. I thought I was helping, but now, with grandchildren of my own, I realise just how much patience he had and the time he spent with me was immensely valuable. I was exposed to farm animal husbandry 'warts and all', not simply the day-to-day tasks of feeding and generally looking after their welfare, which underpins all livestock keeping, but also the more unpleasant aspects such as slaughter.

The farm my grandfather worked on always reared turkeys for the Christmas market and it was his job to kill them. He and his sister, who lived on the farm, then plucked off the feathers and prepared the birds for sale by removing the innards, heads and feet. I remember feeling sad that these birds that I had helped look after were to be killed, but my grandfather helped me understand why this had to be done and that it had to be done humanely.

Looking back at his methods with my current veterinary knowledge, it is clear that improvements could have been made, but it was a humane procedure at that time. My grandfather had a 'killing tree' (my description, not his), on which each turkey was hung upside down by string attached around its legs. The bird then received a heavy blow to its head and neck with a club-shaped piece of wood, which would have effectively rendered it unconscious (stunning as it is referred to today). Then a sharp knife was inserted into its mouth, severing the two carotid arteries, and the bird then effectively bled out. There was always a large amount of blood under the tree and on my grandfather as the bird struggled in its final death throes. This method may seem gruesome by many of today's standards but in my view it was probably as humane a procedure as could have been undertaken at that time.

This same man, who seemed to be able to kill turkeys without showing anything other than humanity to the birds he had to kill, was quite a different man with his pigs. He seemed to genuinely love these animals and I remember him shedding many a tear when they were loaded up and sent off for slaughter.

It was the occasional visit from the local vet, Geoffrey Bowler, however, that cemented my resolve to enter the profession. Geoffrey (or Mr Bowler as my grandfather called him out of respect) was a very striking and dapper gentleman, with a handlebar moustache, bow tie and waistcoat. Whenever he came, my grandfather would make sure he was there and waiting. He would greet Mr Bowler at the car by raising the front of the flat cap he always wore. He would then walk backwards, still lifting the front of his cap, as if he were greeting royalty to the farm. When whatever the procedure he had been called for was complete, a freshly laundered towel, a new bar of soap and a bucket of clean warm water was provided. I often thought of this during my years in practice, as I broke the ice on water troughs to wash my arms after a calving, to then dry them on my trousers or coat. Veterinary life has changed so much, as I hope to explain in the coming chapters.

It seems a very sad admission to make in the 21st century, but two of my hobbies as a boy growing up in the countryside in the 1950s and 1960s were wild flower and birds' egg collecting. I used to ride my bike around the local roads or walk along the hedgerows in pursuit of these hobbies. Wild flowers would be brought back and pressed between sheets of blotting paper and two or more heavy books before being entered into my scrapbook. Birds' egg collecting was a popular pastime when I was young, although I now know that it was illegal to take the eggs of most wild birds even at that time. My school had a large collection of birds' eggs that other pupils and I were asked to sort and categorise in the early 1960s, and we were even given a few spares as a reward for our efforts. It was the Wildlife and Countryside Act 1981, however, that made it illegal to possess or control any wild birds' eggs taken since the original, less restrictive, legislation was made in 1954. I have no idea what happened to the school collection but I know my own was destroyed by mice that gained access to the house. Collecting does still take place but the punishment for breaking the law is now rightly severe, including imprisonment.

My love of wild flowers and my ability to name the majority that I found was to come in useful during my veterinary degree course, as the emphasis moved towards the identification of those that could be toxic to grazing livestock such as bracken, ragwort, hemlock and water dropwort, and trees including yew and laburnum.

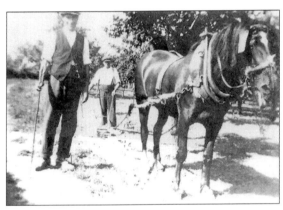

My grandfather Albert Allen, a stockman on a local farm, in the foreground, ploughing with horses.

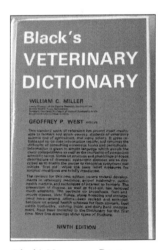

Black's Veterinary Dictionary, a copy of which I had on permanent loan from Evesham library through my teens.

Chapter 4

Pigs, Horses, Goats and Sheep – a Grammar School Education!

I sat and subsequently passed the 11-plus examination in 1960, when I was aged just ten. I still have the letter sent to my parents telling them of my success and I duly started at Prince Henry's Grammar School in Evesham. It seems somewhat ironic in retrospect that the school's acronym of PHGS should be referred to by pupils from the Four Pools County Secondary School in the town as 'Pigs, Horses, Goats and Sheep' in the light of my subsequent career as a farm animal vet!

The daily trip to school started at 8.15am, when the double-decker bus picked me up outside the church for the 25-minute trip into Evesham. The bus carried all secondary school children from the Lench villages but by far the majority (including all my village friends) went to Four Pools on the other side of town. During the next year or so, it was my family (particularly from my father's side, my mother was an only child), from which the majority of the village's grammar school attendees came from. These included my sister, and my cousins Martin and Trevor. It was a salutary message to me that there must have been considerable academic potential in my family through previous generations but because of the the circumstances of the day it was not recognised and nurtured. My sister, my cousins and I were the first generation who had the opportunity to break into the academic stream that leads to university education and beyond, and for that I am eternally grateful. My mother and father must have given me the genes I needed to launch me on my veterinary career.

I began my grammar school life in form 1B, with one of the French teachers, Mr Bradshaw, as my form teacher. I was just ten when I started and I remember struggling a bit in the early years. With hindsight, I now realise that I was suddenly in a pool of pupils who had also passed their 11-plus examination and were, to put it bluntly, a very bright lot. My powers of concentration also were not good.

One of my early reports commented that I seemed to be more fascinated with the trains that ran past the school than I was in learning French. However, when we were all asked what we wanted to be when we grew up, I stated veterinary surgeon amid the usual collection of aspiring teachers, doctors, nurses and engineers. And, yes, we did have one or two who wanted to be train drivers.

I suffered a major setback in my second year when I seriously injured my knee while playing football. Someone fell on the side of my leg when it was outstretched and I clearly remember a searing pain. I was taken to the doctor, who diagnosed a sprain and put a pressure bandage on my badly swollen knee. That night I was in agony and became increasingly delirious. My father, having initially phoned the doctor, decided that I badly needed help and took me to the casualty department in Evesham, where I still remember him carrying me into the waiting room. I was passing out with the pain at that time and was admitted. A large amount of fluid and blood was drawn off the joint and, although I do not know just what the diagnosis was, my parents were told if they had not got me to hospital for treatment that night I could have lost my leg. I remained in hospital for two weeks and wore a full leg plaster for some weeks afterwards. My leg wasted badly and I then had weeks of physiotherapy to rebuild the muscle and get the knee joint to bend again.

As a result, it was decided it would be better for me to repeat my second year and, in retrospect, that was an excellent move since I went from being a struggling pupil and one of the youngest in the class, to a year in which I was a similar age to the others and had already covered much of the syllabus. This was undoubtedly the time I began to set a foundation for my future career aspirations.

I also developed a real interest in athletics, winning the school and then South Worcestershire schools 220-yard title. I eventually got into the Worcestershire schools athletics team and represented my county at 220 yards in the All England Championships. Despite being only just over 5 ft 8 in tall, I also developed an uncanny ability in the high jump. I broke the school record of 5 ft 4 in and eventually cleared 5 ft 9 in, effectively jumping more than my own height, using the 'straddle' technique into a sandpit.

During my time as a pupil, Prince Henry's Grammar School had around 700 pupils and was a very traditional co-educational establishment with a very strict regime. The headmaster, Mr Miller, and headmistress, Mrs Dean, were both highly respected by both pupils and staff alike, but Mr Miller in particular was a fearsome character who never stood for any misbehaviour. He only had to open the door leading from his office into the old hall thoroughfare area to cause everyone to freeze to the spot and look away, hoping he would not target one of them for having dirty shoes, an untidy uniform or long hair. I never saw myself as a rebel but I was picked out on more than one occasion for having long or unruly hair. I complained to my parents but both of them agreed with Mr Miller and I was sent straight to the hairdresser. I only found myself outside his study on one occasion, when a group of us were sent together for rowdy behaviour and ignoring the attempts of a prefect to quieten us down during a wet playtime indoors. To heighten our fears, we were sent individually, not as a group – a hard lesson learned!

As a teenage boy, I suppose one of my lasting memories of Mrs Dean, who was an excellent mathematics teacher, was fairly predictable. During my time at Prince Henry's, the hemline of the girls' dresses was visibly rising as the miniskirt became ever more fashionable. There was a strict uniform code, with a specific number of inches specified as the distance between knee and hem. Any girl who was spotted with a skirt that seemed to be shorter than the regulation length was sent to the headmistress. It did not matter if Mrs Dean was in the middle of a maths lesson, the poor girl was made to kneel upright on a desk at the front of the mixed sex class while the skirt length was measured. It was a fairly regular but quite welcome distraction for us teenage boys. This would never be allowed to happen today and reminds me of a much later humiliation of fellow female students that occurred at the Royal Veterinary College during freshers' week that I will describe later.

There were four houses at Prince Henry's and each pupil was allocated to one on their first day, a system that reminds me of Hogwarts in the Harry Potter stories. The selection was fairly random and was often linked to which house your older sibling was already in. I was in Lichfield house, of which I was eventually made captain in my final year. The other houses were Holland, Workman and Deacle. There was a very active and competitive inter-house spirit during my time at the school, with most activities scoring points towards the eventual annual award of the shield to the top house.

This competitiveness was mainly focused on sporting activities, such as inter-house football, rugby and hockey and netball tournaments, but also included individual points scored for positions gained in the annual cross-country race and athletics sports days. There was a wide range of other activities that counted towards house points, including music and singing competitions and poetry recitations.

I sometimes look back on these activities and compare them with school pursuits today. I vividly remember compulsory cross-country runs undertaken in all weathers and you had to have a very valid excuse not to take part. Once, after a long spell of very heavy rain, the river Avon was flooded and had broken its banks. It was cross-country day, however, and we were sent off on a course that took us down to Offenham Ferry, where we had to run through what was usually a narrow stream that fed the Avon. On this occasion we had to wade through flowing water that was waist high and very cold. It was character building, perhaps, but undoubtedly something that would never be sanctioned under today's health and safety culture.

One compulsory part of the school curriculum for boys was the Combined Cadet Force (CCF) and I hated it! On one day each week for a number of years we all had to wear armed forces, usually army, uniform to school. This included a black beret and heavy, shiny boots. There were many days when I turned up at the village bus stop as the sole pupil in uniform. I felt so self-conscious and I became the subject of ridicule by pupils from the secondary school until I got off the bus, when many of them saluted. We had to wear this uniform all morning during lessons and then finished with marching and other drill activities later in the day. There were also regular uniform inspections. I was so relieved when I eventually reached the age when the CCF was no longer compulsory and I never had to wear that uniform again.

Prince Henry's was renowned as being a very good school when I was a pupil and still is today, although it is no longer a grammar school. It is now known as Prince Henry's High School, a secondary school with academy status. It remains a co-educational school but has increased dramatically in size, with around 1,260 students aged between 13 and 18.

As I moved towards the fifth form (now referred to as year 11), my O-level choices became tailored towards my career choice, which remained veterinary surgeon. I took and passed nine O-levels: English language, English literature, French, Latin, geography, mathematics, physics, chemistry and biology. My choice for A-levels seemed obvious and I then embarked on my final hurdle before applying to university, namely getting good pass levels in chemistry, biology and physics. The A-level requirements for entry on to the veterinary course today have changed dramatically. When I applied, it was almost unthinkable to select any subjects other than the three I had chosen, although mathematics was an option some students could choose. Today, I interview prospective undergraduates at my former place of study, the Royal Veterinary College, and one of its primary objectives is to attract the all-round student. Those called for interview still possess A-levels with a scientific bias but often also have studied a variety of subjects, including languages and humanities.

I eventually achieved three A-level passes, with an A in chemistry and B grades in biology and physics.

In my final year, the school decided to put me forward to sit the Oxbridge entrance exams, specifically for Cambridge which hosts one of the UK veterinary colleges. These are sat before A-levels and in retrospect gave me a head start in my revision programme. I was successful and was called for interview at Downing College, Cambridge. I had not long passed my driving test but borrowed the family car, an Austin A40, to drive myself there. It was an interview over two days, beginning with dinner alongside other potential undergraduates and staff members, and followed by a fairly gruelling interview the next day. I was unsuccessful and realised that I had found myself totally outside my comfort zone. I was a country boy who had only very rarely left his village roots, and Cambridge at the time seemed very elitist. Part of me wishes that I had been successful but I also recognise that I may well have found life at Cambridge during the early 1970s to be very difficult and, I suspect, very expensive.

The choice of which universities to apply to when filling out my University and Colleges Admission Service (UCAS) application form was relatively straightforward in that I chose five of the six UK universities then offering a veterinary degree course, namely Cambridge, Bristol, London, Glasgow and Edinburgh. As my final choice I plumped for University College London to study human medicine. I'm not sure why I didn't choose Liverpool as I now know the veterinary school very well, having lectured there regularly over the past few years. My choice of a medical degree may seem an odd one but at that time it had an easier A-level entry requirement than those of the veterinary schools and was essentially my fallback option.

Interestingly, it was my father who had some reservations about my pursuit of veterinary medicine as a career because it appeared not to have the kudos that it perhaps enjoys today. He had always harboured ambitions for me to become either a doctor or a lawyer, although he was committed totally to supporting my eventual route into the veterinary world and, in his own quiet way, was proud of my later achievements. I'm not sure I would have made a good doctor and my wife Gerry, who has worked in the health sector all her working life, agrees!

These days, prior to gaining entry on to the veterinary course, prospective undergraduates have to demonstrate their commitment, in addition to gaining the necessary academic qualifications. The system is now very structured and, although requirements do vary from college to college, essentially prospective undergraduates have to demonstrate an 'experience portfolio'. This must include the names and addresses of veterinary practices they have spent time with, together with what is expected to be a wide range of other experiences such as helping on farms milking cows, lambing, working with horses, helping to muck out stables, working in kennels or walking dogs.

Having had the opportunity to read many personal statements of prospective undergraduates I interview, it never ceases to amaze me just how widespread these experiences can be. I have interviewed candidates who have helped out at open farms, pets corners in zoos, pet shops, riding for the disabled centres, guide dog kennels and alpaca farms. Indeed, one memorable candidate presented me with a dissertation she had prepared for the interview on the mating behaviour of alpacas.

When I was preparing to apply there were no such rigid requirements but there was nevertheless an expectation that the candidate could demonstrate commitment in an interview.

I already had a fair amount of experience with poultry as we kept them at home; with pigs and cattle that my grandfather was responsible for; and with my own pet rabbits and our cats. I spent some time with Wilf Major helping him to milk the cows and generally learning about their care. My grandfather and I both mentioned my interest to Mr Bowler, who then invited me to spend some time at his practice in Evesham. This was my golden opportunity, which I grabbed with both hands, and I spent many Saturday mornings and much of my holiday time at the practice, thinking nothing of the ten-mile round trip on my bike to get there and back.

The practice, which is still there today, was based at Merstow Green in Evesham and was mixed, meaning that it dealt with a wide range of animals including farm animals, pets and horses. All those working there made me feel very welcome and in time I became a very junior member of the team – unpaid, of course.

The best part of this experience was the time I actually spent with the vets themselves. I was taken out on calls by Mr Bowler and his partner, Roger Martin. I was able to watch at first-hand what an important role the farm vet played in maintaining the health and welfare (and profitability) of the farms they were visiting. Much of what I saw would be considered routine, such as disbudding calves (destroying the bud from which the horn grows by thermocautery), dehorning older cattle (literally removing the horns under anaesthetic, usually with a saw or wire) and castrating male calves.

At that time in the 1960s, we had far less tuberculosis (TB) in cattle than we have now, with the UK being virtually free of the disease. However, routine tuberculin testing was still carried out to monitor herds for new infection. My role at the time was to sit on (usually) a straw bale, recording, in a notebook, skin measurements which would denote whether or not the test was positive or negative. To the best of my knowledge, I never came across a positive case; all farms in the Evesham area at that time were free of infection. Looking back at that time, however, makes one realise just how dynamic disease can be, particularly with reference to bovine TB. I have witnessed a gradual progression in the sophistication of tests and testing procedures available to the modern veterinary surgeon; yet despite this, there has been a gradual increase in the level of TB in the UK cattle population, to its current high level. Admittedly there are a number of factors that have and are still playing their part in this increase, but it is of significance that we are still applying the same comparative skin test that I watched a veterinary surgeon using in the 1960s. TB is a complex disease, and the immune response elicited following infection is not a simple one that we can assess using currently established serological tests. At the time of writing, however, real progress is being made in the development of dedicated blood tests for TB in camelids and goats, which in due course may also become available for use in cattle – although current legislation that is based on the use of the comparative skin test will need to be changed.

Back in the practice, I was present during the daily surgeries. I watched the vets deal with a succession of worried owners with their pets, mainly dogs and cats, that had problems still dealt with by modern veterinary practitioners such as itchy skin, bad ears, cuts and bite wounds. There was also the daily operations list of cat and bitch spays and castrations and broken legs to repair, all of which again I was able to observe.

This further consolidated my resolve to become a vet, particularly as in the Evesham practice there was no real specialism. Every vet was a jack of all trades, moving with effortless ease (at least in my eyes) from a lame cow to a ewe that needed lambing, from a worried owner with a budgerigar to spaying a bitch. They were true general practitioners and this became my goal.

In return for the experience I was gaining, it was expected that I would provide whatever help was needed around the practice. I soon became adept at washing up the instruments after operations, cleaning out kennels, washing down tables between consultations and exercising dogs. In time, I progressed to being able to assist in operations, such as holding instruments, and restraining dogs or cats for the induction of anaesthesia or for euthanasia. This was all good experience.

Interviews were rarely undertaken when I applied to university back in the late 1960s and, apart from Cambridge, I only had one further interview, at Glasgow. This seemed an awfully long way from Church Lench at that time but I was fortunate to have a fellow pupil at Prince Henry's who had also applied there to study veterinary medicine and who by chance also had an interview on the same day. We travelled together by train on Sunday afternoon, ready for our interviews on Monday. It was the first time either of us had travelled so far without our parents and we were slightly apprehensive about the journey and getting around Glasgow, in addition to our concerns about the interview itself.

We arrived on a cold dark, damp and very foggy night during either January or February. As we came out of Glasgow station to find a taxi to take us to our hotel, we noticed some police activity and a man lying on the pavement with what appeared to be blood nearby. The taxi driver merely shrugged his shoulders and stated: 'He's probably been stabbed, it happens around here'. To this day, I think that the cold, the thick fog and the stabbing were the reasons I turned down the offer made to me by Glasgow University. Again, I have lectured at the city's veterinary college for the past few years and I have nothing but respect for its course and location.

I got only one further offer, from the Royal Veterinary College (RVC), part of London University, and I accepted it. I began the course in October 1969.

The RVC was founded in 1791 and is the oldest and largest of the UK veterinary schools. It became a college of the University of London in 1949.

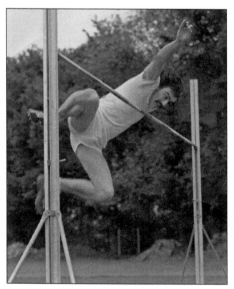

Me breaking the school high jump record at 5 feet 9 inches.

Chapter 5
How Veterinary College Life has Changed!

I embarked on the veterinary degree course with some savings built up from my fruit picking skills and a full grant from Worcestershire Education Authority. There were no course fees at that time and my day-to-day living expenses, including accommodation, books and other necessities, were all just about covered by my grant. That meant I didn't have to rely on my parents and, more importantly, I did not leave at the end of five years with a massive burden of debt. That was a major difference from the current situation faced by modern veterinary undergraduates. This changing world to which I keep referring has now resulted in course fees of £9,000 a year, limited access to public funding and debts on qualification of an average of £50,000, and in many cases much more.

The veterinary undergraduates of today have an increased financial burden, partly due to their course lasting five years and not the average three. This burden is compounded by the need from year one to gain experience on farms and the expectation that undergraduates will work alongside vets (so called EMS or extra-mural study) during holiday time, thus leaving limited opportunity for temporary employment and a chance to earn some money.

First year students were encouraged to live in halls of residence, rather than move into flats and bedsits, and I applied for accommodation in Commonwealth Hall, in Cartwright Gardens, WC1, a building that is still in use and looks relatively unchanged from the outside 40 years after I left. It was one of three, adjoining, multi-faculty University of London halls situated opposite gardens in this rather elegant crescent. There has been one major change in the past 40 years: during my time there, between 1969 and 1971, Commonwealth Hall was male-only. Next door was Canterbury Hall, which at that time was a female-only hall, and next door again was Hughes Parry Hall, again all male. All now have mixed sex intakes.

When the day came to move down to London, the family car was packed with all my worldly goods, which were mainly clothes, shoes, toiletries, food (including a box of pears), my radio and an old-fashioned spool-to-spool tape recorder on which I had recorded music from the radio. Since then, I have moved my daughters back and forth from their respective universities many times and it is obvious that today's student needs far more, including computers, scanners, printers and music systems. As a result, I needed a bigger car!

My father had never previously driven in London and neither had I, but with the confidence of youth and without the aid of satnav, we set off for Commonwealth Hall. I drove, my father sat in the front navigating and my mother was in the back completely surrounded by my belongings. Admittedly, there was much less traffic in 1969, and it was also a Sunday, but we made it. I was allocated room 3.20, on the third floor and facing into the central courtyard of the building. Once settled in, I then drove my parents to Hanger Lane on the A40 back towards Evesham, where my father took over to drive home. I caught the tube back to central London and my university life began.

Being part of a multi-faculty hall was an excellent introduction to college life and most of the early socialising within Commonwealth was done during meal times. Within a short time, we established a table consisting regularly of two other vet students, one dental student and one law student, with three others studying English, geography and biology. We all remained friends throughout my two years in Commonwealth.

The following day was Monday and my first day as a veterinary undergraduate. I had studied my A to Z of London and knew more or less where the RVC was located. I came out of the doors of Commonwealth wearing my green and white college scarf at almost the same time as another student wearing an identical one. It quickly became clear that we were heading in the same direction and with one question, 'Vet school?' I met the first of my fellow students, called Jan.

He was from Maesycwmmer in south Wales, a miner's son, and now a well-known and highly respected equine vet. Our first obstacle was to cross the busy Euston Road before heading first north along Ossulston Street, then into Charrington Street, then across Crowndale Road past the College Arms pub (now replaced by flats) and St Pancras Hospital and into Royal College Street. The RVC was a few hundred yards along on the right.

There were two major differences between my first year RVC intake and the first year intake of today. To begin with, my year had 65 undergraduates, compared with 250 today. But whereas my year had 59 men and 6 women, around 90 per cent of today's intake is female. The feminisation of the veterinary profession has been steadily increasing, over the past 10 to 15 years in particular, and many possible reasons for this have been proposed. Female students will tell you they are much more intelligent, and this may be true, but interestingly it isn't simply that more female students are getting the grades required for vet school entry, there are actually more applying and the ratio of total applicants to successful ones is very similar between males and females. Rather, it appears that young women are choosing veterinary medicine as a career in far greater numbers than men. This trend is also apparent in the hospital medical course intake, and as a result the medical profession is also becoming more female dominated.

The first few days of my course were taken up with introductory talks, familiarisation with the building, kitting out with laboratory coats and being given our list of required textbooks. In addition, there was freshers' week, which was partly intended to integrate us into RVC college student life (particularly how we stood up to the RVC Yard of Ale competition), but also, as the college was part of London University, it gave me the opportunity to join a wide number of different clubs and societies.

Part of this initiation week was taken up with the selection of Miss Fresher by a process which, with hindsight, makes me cringe with embarrassment. This is partly due to my participation with all the other male students from across the five years but mainly because of my recollection of what my female fresher undergraduate colleagues were persuaded to do. As this was a veterinary college, and as livestock shows were part of the agricultural landscape, these poor girls were made to parade up and down a walkway built across tables in the refectory to be 'judged' by us males on the basis of the amount of applause or wolf whistles each one received. I'm pleased to say that this tradition has now died out, predominantly as a result of the dramatic change in male-to-female ratios. Perhaps the situation should now be reversed?

During the first year, or pre-clinical year one, most of my time was spent in Camden Town studying predominantly anatomy, physiology and biochemistry. I was also introduced to the subject of animal husbandry, a discipline that covers nutrition, housing design, basic management and breeding principles across all species. Much of this latter part of the course was spent out at the RVC field station at Hawkshead and at Boltons Park, a working, mixed farm, both of which were in the Potters Bar area of Hertfordshire. Both still exist, but Hawkshead is now a very large modern site, having undergone massive development and investment as the major RVC teaching facility, and also includes the purpose-built Queen Mother Hospital for Small Animals. The only part of the campus I still recognise is totally surrounded by new buildings, while the lecture theatre we used is now a gym and coffee shop.

One major difference between the way I was taught in the pre-clinical years and the teaching of today is simply how separate the pre-clinical and clinical teaching was during my undergraduate years. I learned anatomy for two years, then spent a year forgetting much of it, before beginning to realise why I needed to know it when learning pathology in my third year and surgery in my final year. Today's student is taught anatomy in year one (as I was), but alongside this purely discipline teaching is an indication throughout as to why certain structures are important for later use in clinical subjects, such as anaesthesia and surgery.

Anatomy teaching was a combination of lectures and practical classes including basic cell structure, histology (essentially studying each body system in microscopic detail) and gross anatomy, considering organ structure and, in particular, the differences between the wide range of species covered in the course. The kidney of a cow, for example, is very different in structure to the kidney of a sheep. Practical sessions were divided into live anatomy demonstrations and morbid dissection classes. I took the opportunity 39 years after I left the RVC to revisit these two demonstration areas and, to my surprise, they had changed very little in basic structure, despite massive change around the remainder of the Camden and Hawkshead sites. Looking back, I suspect that they had not changed much in the years leading up to my arrival as an undergraduate.

Live anatomy demonstrations gave students the opportunity to palpate the body of a live dog, cat, sheep or cow, learning how to identify key structures in the musculo-skeletal system and internal body organs by feel.

During dissection classes using smaller species, we were divided into groups of four, depending on our position in the alphabet. My team of four included Robin, Richard and Jenny. We began with a cat, then progressed to a greyhound. All cadavers were fixed in formol saline to preserve them and prevent decay so that we could work on them over a number of weeks. This illustrates another change in attitude encompassed by modern health and safety concerns. Today, we handle formol saline under strict containment, mainly in safety cabinets. Any spills are considered as potentially serious incidents; staff must evacuate the area and a clean-up must be undertaken by staff wearing full respiratory and eye protection. There is now plenty of evidence to suggest that formalin fumes can be hazardous, and the approaches that we adopt today quite rightly protect the individual working in such an environment. No such precautions were taken during our afternoon-long dissection classes, other than having extractor fans switched on – making the room very cold during winter (another health and safety factor considered today). We dissected until we could no longer see clearly as our eyes (and noses) began to run profusely due to the exposure to formalin fumes. After turning away for a few minutes – and after our eyes cleared – we could resume our examinations. Whilst fully appreciating and supporting the current need to have a clear health and safety policy in place for anyone working or studying in an area in which exposure to formalin fumes is a possibility, I can't help thinking back to those dissection days. It never seemed to do any lasting harm, and none of us ever left the dissection room with a stuffy head cold – nasal chambers and sinuses were always clear!

We mainly took it in turns to dissect whatever it was we were studying that day, and were mindful of the need to do it well for the benefit of the remainder of the group. However, Robin, a larger than life character, had a phrase that I still remember so well: 'If in doubt, cut it out'. We did lose a number of vital structures we were supposed to find and study to the bin as a result of his enthusiasm. When we moved on to dissect an adult cow and horse this was mainly undertaken by one of the anatomy lecturers demonstrating to groups of us gathered around.

We veterinary students and my hall friend Geraint, studying dentistry, all dissected on the same days, so meal times were mainly spent comparing experiences with our greyhound and Geraint's head and neck dissection. We were often left alone on the meal table after our non-medical undergraduate colleagues had left in disgust.

Art, and drawing in particular, has never come easily to me but at that time it was our main method of recording what we were seeing. I lacked the ability to transfer a three-dimensional image on to paper, particularly when such drawings were part of later exam questions. I had to remember where and how the lines had been drawn as I could never visualise the image in my mind and transfer it to the exam paper. Today's students have an array of digital cameras, smartphones and tablets, all capable of taking high-resolution photographs that can be easily stored and studied later. I have demonstrated post-mortem techniques to many students during my career but this approach of photographing everything is now clearly in evidence as students click away around me.

My first textbook purchase at Foyle's in Charing Cross Road was a copy of Sisson and Grossman's *The Anatomy of the Domestic Animals,* a book that 40 years later I still have on my bookshelf and have referred to many times over the years. I started my anatomy course with a book I had brought with me from school. I had been awarded the Aldrich Prize for Chemistry and Physics during my final year and chose *Schaffer's Essentials of Histology* as my prize. Sadly this was a medical text and of limited value on my veterinary course but that copy also still sits on my bookshelf.

Physiology, the biological study of the functions of living organisms and their parts, was also a subject taught by a combination of lectures and practical sessions. One memorable part of the course was studying skeletal and cardiac muscle function, mainly using frog muscle. We used kymograph drums, devices that graphically record changes in position over time via a stylus and which are most commonly used to record changes in pressure or motion. The kymograph consists of a drum to which the stylus is attached, recording the changes on to paper wrapped around the drum and covered in carbon by holding it over a lighted candle, the stylus making a mark through the carbon. The equipment would be attached to the piece of muscle under study and the smoked drum paper trace could be 'fixed' so it could be stored for later study.

All the pre-clinical teaching is essential to form the foundation to the clinical years, the adage 'you have to understand the normal to appreciate the abnormal' can never be more true than in a veterinary degree course. That said, we all yearned to move on to what can only be referred to as 'real vetting'. The animal husbandry component was just that. We learned the principles of building design and ventilation, breeds of the different farm animals and feeding principles both in theory and practical ration formulation.

This teaching was not simply confined to farm animals. We also considered the proper management of dogs and cats, including how to feed and house them, and horses, including their complex markings based on hair whorls and correct colour description. We were also taught the different types of harness, bridles and bits as well as farriery – the art of shoeing a horse. In addition, we were shown how to age horses and other farm livestock by their teeth, looking at numbers of teeth, eruption and growth rates, tooth wear and loss and more specific pointers such as Galvayne's groove. This groove is located on the lateral surface of the upper third incisor in horses and appears first near the gum line at about ten years of age. The groove extends halfway down the tooth at 15 years and all the way down by 20 years. By approximately 25 years, Galvayne's groove is half gone, and by 30 years it has disappeared completely. An invaluable source of this very practical information is the textbook *Practical Animal Husbandry* by Miller and Robertson, now out of print and highly sought after. I still have my copy and have used it on many occasions since qualifying, particularly the sections on teeth eruption which is often an important factor in ageing carcasses for forensic examination, an area in which I became skilled later in my career.

The 65 students who started at the RVC came from a wide demographic background, brought together by an ambition to be a veterinary surgeon and having achieved the high academic qualifications required for entry. There were obviously many strengths and weaknesses that became apparent. I had grown up in the country, had spent much of my formative time with my grandfather on the farm, and knew a fair bit about livestock management. The differences in our backgrounds first became apparent to me when Tony, Dave and I were together on the farm one day, when Tony asked me what the difference was between two stacks of bales in one of the buildings. 'Why is one called hay and the other straw? they both look the same to me', he asked. I explained that hay is meadow grass cut and dried in the field and used mainly as a feed for livestock, whereas straw is made from the stems of cereals such as wheat and barley as it is harvested. It is of much lower nutritional value and used mainly as bedding.

My main animal husbandry weakness was with horses. Although I had walked alongside my grandfather and his horses as a small child, I had never ridden and knew little about the animals' daily management, in particular how to handle them. Together with about ten other students from my year, I signed up for a series of ten riding lessons at a local stable at Patchetts Green, now a thriving equestrian centre. During these sessions we learned how to put on a saddle and bridle in addition to learning to ride. It was a pastime I never really took to, although the lessons I learned and the confidence I gained in handling horses were invaluable. I never really did any serious horse veterinary work during my career but one student, Jan – whom I met on my first day – also learned to ride at Patchetts Green and is now an eminent equine veterinary surgeon.

We seemed to have far more examinations during my time at the RVC than modern students but I suppose I would say that – it's like saying O- and A-levels were much harder than modern GCSEs. One thing I did notice when at the RVC recently is that each student now has a number, which presumably only they know. When results go up on the noticeboard now you can remain anonymous, as your mark will only be recorded alongside your number. In my day, results went up with our names alongside. Most results would be posted in alphabetical order but there were some occasions when they were put in mark order with the highest at the top and the lowest at the bottom. I clearly remember looking at such a list with increasing anxiety as my eyes scanned down towards the lower end. I never finished bottom but the occasional exam did see me placed lower than I would have wished, mainly because of poor revision.

We invariably had one or more three-hour written papers for each discipline, coupled with practical exams. The latter were often referred to as a steeplechase as they tended to consist of a number of stations, each with a set question and a designated time in which to answer it. At the time limit, a bell would ring and we would move round in rotation until all the questions had been answered. They were designed to test our powers of observation and reasoning under pressure. Such tests might involve a piece of tissue such as a kidney for which we had to identify which species it came from, and a diagram of its ultrastructure to test our ability to identify specific parts of the organ. There might have been a bone with a small area coloured red and the question might have been: 'What muscle attaches to this area? or a skull with a small hole highlighted with the question: 'Name two structures that pass through this hole'.

I passed my pre-clinical final exams at the end of my second year and moved on to the second part of the course, when the real veterinary work would begin.

Living in WC1 was a great experience. I could walk to Tottenham Court Road in around 10 to 15 minutes and the West End was close by. I did not have my car with me for the first two years, mainly due to problems finding a parking space, but as the course was almost entirely based in Camden Town, within walking distance of my hall, it was not a problem. I travelled out to the farm and field station by bus. The local tube station was Russell Square, only a five to ten-minute walk from the hall of residence and public transport was much cheaper in comparison to today's prices, so travelling around was very easy.

A number of my friends in the early years came from Wales and at weekends I became an honorary Welsh citizen. As such, I spent many Saturday evenings in the Prince of Wales pub in Covent Garden, although at this time I wasn't really a practised bitter drinker and, although I learned very quickly, I was often referred to as a lightweight by my more experienced Welsh drinking friends.

The RVC was a small college but being part of London University gave me the option to visit many other colleges for their social events. One problem at that time, with 59 males and only 6 females in our year, came during RVC social events, many of which quickly descended into drinking competitions complete with raucous singing. There were occasions, however, when there was a need for more female company, so invites to our dances went to our twin college, University College Hospital Medical School, and specifically to the nurses who worked in the hospital a stone's throw from the college. In later years, when I was out at Hawkshead, the same dilemma was solved by inviting female students from the local teacher training college to attend and at least one student in my year met his wife on one of these visits.

Some of us also saw an advert or flyer advertising free haircuts at the London College of Fashion in Oxford Circus. A few of us went along mainly to invite the girls to our social events but also to get a free haircut. It was quite interesting how the frequency of haircuts went up among us, as a visit to what was a very attractive group of young women was quite an incentive.

We did not have the resources to attract the big name bands and singers who played regularly at the other, larger colleges, but I remember the Nashville Teens played at the Camden campus one year. One band not too well known at the time, and hence cheap, that we did hire was Kilburn and the High Roads, who were formed by Ian Dury in 1970. They split up in 1979 when Dury left to form what would become his better-known group, The Blockheads. It was much easier to get tickets to concerts in the early 1970s and queuing usually resulted in success. This is in marked contrast to today's ticket allocation, which is often gone in minutes via the internet. During my time at the RVC in central London I saw Simon and Garfunkel at the Albert Hall and Emerson, Lake and Palmer on several occasions, including a concert with the London Symphony Orchestra at the Royal Festival Hall. I remember seeing Deep Purple with the Royal Philharmonic, again at the Albert Hall, and Curved Air at the Royal Festival Hall. I also saw Hawkwind at the London School of Economics, a very psychedelic show and what I believe was my first experience of passive cannabis smoking.

One artist I felt I almost grew up with was Elton John. I first saw him playing his piano and singing alone in the refectory at University College Hospital Medical School on a Saturday evening. One year later, when I was revising in the newly-built Euston Library/Shaw Theatre complex, I heard what sounded like Elton's first hit *Your Song* being played very loudly. It transpired he was rehearsing in the Shaw and I managed to slip into the back and watch. He played a concert there that night and, although we didn't get tickets, it was loud enough that we could stand outside and listen. The following year Elton had progressed to playing at the Royal Festival Hall and then on to Hammersmith Odeon for what became his traditional Christmas parties. I kept many of my concert tickets pinned to the noticeboard in my room, including one for the Elton John and London Symphony Orchestra concert at the Royal Festival Hall from 3 March 1971. I sat in row M, seat 22, and the ticket cost me 18 shillings (90p was printed in brackets as the country became familiar with decimalisation). To my surprise, I sold this used ticket on eBay 42 years later to a collector for around £30. I only wish I hadn't thrown out my other used ticket stubs.

It was at the Euston Library/Shaw Theatre complex where I met my first wife, Diane. Gail, my girlfriend from my home area, had effectively dumped me, mainly due to the fact I came home only twice during my first term. I was revising for my end of year exams and Diane was revising for her exams at Parliament Hill School. I felt an immediate attraction to her, with her long hair cascading down her back and, having exchanged notes, we eventually met in the café, whereupon I plucked up the courage to ask her out. We eventually married prior to me joining the final year. Diane lived at 5 Mornington Crescent and I became a regular visitor.

As I stated earlier, Commonwealth was a men-only hall and any visitor of either sex had to sign in to gain access to the student rooms. Diane was my first serious girlfriend in London and became a regular visitor. There was a strict policy, however, that guests had to leave the building by 11.30pm and overnight stays were not allowed. If your visitor had not signed out, then there was a knock on your door as midnight approached. We found ways around this by helping each other out and forging leaving signatures.

During my second year in hall, I moved to the seventh floor, specifically room 7.07, and my window looked out towards Russell Square. I had a very clear view of the North Sea Fish Restaurant in Leigh Street below, which is still serving fish and chips 40 years later. I could watch the queue from my window and plan my run down to join it if I were hungry. I was also introduced to squash in Commonwealth Hall, a game I continued to play for many years until the body became too old. There were two squash courts in the basement and a group of us decided to try our hand at the game, which I quickly took to once I had got used to the much smaller racket head and rubber ball. I had played tennis at school and had also spent hours banging a tennis ball against the side of our house back in Church Lench. It must have driven my mother mad at the time as the kitchen was the other side of the wall but it was similar to squash and perhaps why I took to it instantly. A group of us also used to go out for runs around nearby Regent's Park late at night. Jan and I had both been successful athletes before coming to London, although he was a distance runner and I was a sprinter so I did struggle a bit to keep up with him. We both wore our tracksuits emblazoned with the badges we had won. I had my Worcestershire county badge and proudly wore my two Amateur Athletic Association graded badges.

As a student at the RVC in Camden Town, I enjoyed complimentary entry into London Zoo in Regent's Park for study purposes. In fact, it was a really good way of impressing prospective girlfriends whom you could get in free through a dedicated entrance at the north of the zoo. Diane and I spent many days there.

Although small, the RVC did play its part in charity fundraising and rag weeks, and two such ventures proved to be great fun. The first was an inter-year model animal push from the RVC through central London to Wye College in Kent. I cannot remember our actual animal, but it was made from wire mesh covered in papier mâché and, of course, it had a large phallus. Starting in the early hours of the morning to satisfy the police instructions to clear London as soon as possible, we pushed our respective models on wheels, finishing in at the school of agriculture in Wye for a social evening. The second fundraiser involved pushing a wheelbarrow full of elephant dung we had acquired from London Zoo to the Bristol University site at Langford, where it was used to plant a tree. For the record, I pushed for two sections across Salisbury Plain.

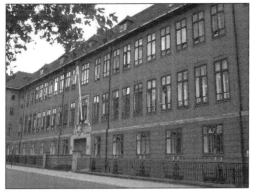

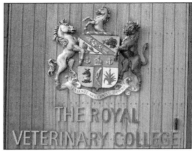

Royal Veterinary College coat of arms at the Hawkshead campus.

Royal Veterinary College in Camden Town, London.

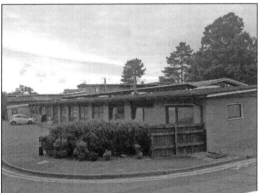

The 'old part' of the Hawkshead campus photographed in 2014, now enveloped by the new modern buildings as the site has been enhanced.

An Elton John ticket for a concert I attended in 1971, sold as a collectors item in 2013!

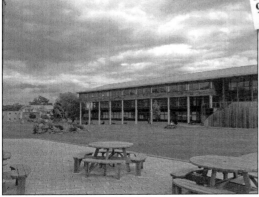

Some of the new buildings on the Hawkshead campus photographed in 2014.

Chapter 6
Do I Really Need to Know All This?

At last the clinical years began and, with them, a move out of central London and life in a hall of residence. Five of us decided to share a house at the start of our third year and as more of the course time would now be spent in Hawkshead rather than Camden, we settled on a three-storey house in Holly Park Road, Friern Barnet, in north London. Also sharing to make up the six required to pay the rent was a friend of Dave who worked in the insurance business. Our first task was to draw lots for bedrooms, as at least two people would have to share a room. I drew the small backwards facing bedroom on the middle floor and was disappointed at first, but at least it was quiet and private.

We had a communal kitchen and, although we did eat takeaways and fish and chips together occasionally, none of us was a keen enough chef to take the lead so we all tended to do our own thing. Visiting girlfriends were always welcome to help feed us. The buttery at Hawkshead was a fallback for a cooked meal at lunchtime, with perhaps the least imaginative menu I have ever come across. Your choice each day was either pie and baked beans or pasty and baked beans.

The third year was free of the really important section exams and, although term time tests were a regular feature, these were not used in your final assessment as they tend to be in the continual assessment course of today. With us, it was an all-or-nothing performance in the sector exams referred to as first BVetMed and second BVetMed, leading up to the award of your BVetMed (Bachelor of Veterinary Medicine) degree after four years and two terms.

Living in a house free of the restrictions of halls of residence was an experience and we made the most of it. We all became hooked on the board game Risk and spent many evenings sitting around playing it. We had a small television with three channels, a world away from the Sky, Virgin and other TV packages that seem to be a necessity in student accommodation today. Also, there were obviously no PCs or handheld games consoles. Risk may sound dull to today's student but we had some really good raucous evenings around the board.

Parties were also now permitted as we had our own space and understanding neighbours. This was the era of the Party Four and Party Seven Watneys Red Barrel beer containers and I can still remember the different methods for getting them open – and the mess made by the beer escaping under pressure!

I also had my Mini up in London at that time and it is quite amusing in retrospect to recall how many students I could cram into such a small car.

During my fourth year, in which my second BVetMed exams were to take place, I decided to move into a bedsit to allow me to focus more on my studies with fewer distractions. This basement in a house in Hamilton Park in Highbury was probably the worst accommodation I had during my time in London. Next door in the other basement bedsit was Richard, another student from my year, and we met up regularly and discussed coursework. This accommodation was within a few hundred yards of the old Arsenal football stadium and I could easily hear the crowd on match days. I knew the number of goals scored from the sounds but not necessarily the actual scores for either team.

I continued my relationship with Diane throughout these years and she became a regular visitor to both properties, even introducing some of her female friends to my fellow students. One of them, Christine, eventually married one of my housemates, Gordon.

The third and fourth years gave us an introduction to the more clinical parts of the course – the main two modules were pathology and animal husbandry – and we began to get to grips with medicine, surgery, anaesthesia and pharmacology.

The teaching staff at the RVC contained some of the most eminent veterinary surgeons of their day and it was a privilege to have been taught by a number of them, some of whom were at the pinnacle of their careers during my time at the college, while others were on the rise.

The former category included Professor Hancock (anatomy); Professor Jukes (physiology); Professor Cotchin (pathology); Professor Formston (surgery); Professor Arthur (obstetrics); and Professor Bell (medicine), all of whom were recognised for their eminence and respected by us all. On the way up were Barry Edwards (surgery) and David Noakes (obstetrics).

Pathology was a discipline I really enjoyed during my time at the RVC and, oddly enough, was the field I eventually worked in until my retirement after my first nine years as a practitioner. I believe much of my enthusiasm came from the excellent teaching I had within the department of pathology, particularly from its head, Professor Cotchin. He was a true gentleman and an inspiring lecturer. He was very quiet, yet authoritative, someone who earned our respect, not demanded it. If a particular topic was unclear even to one student who asked a question, it was never that student who was at fault. Instead, Professor Cotchin shouldered the blame for not making his point easier to understand.

Pathology was broken down into a number of component parts, each of which was studied in its own right. The disciplines covered included morbid or gross pathology, histopathology and cellular pathology, bacteriology, virology, parasitology and immunology. Having had personal involvement with many of these disciplines in my career as a veterinary investigation officer, I have seen many changes in the way they have evolved from what I was taught because of our increased knowledge. Pathology may not have advanced to the degree that medicine and surgery have but considerable progress has been made.

Professor Cotchin and his colleagues in the gross pathology, morbid anatomy and histopathology/cellular pathology disciplines taught us by both lecture and practical lessons. The practical sessions were more focused on the cellular components of pathology – effectively spending long periods looking down the microscope – than on gross pathology. I recognise that to become a specialist pathologist requires skills in both disciplines but as the majority of us were heading towards veterinary practice it was the ability to undertake post-mortem examination and recognise gross changes of disease that I personally found to be lacking. Most of us will have rarely spent much time with a microscope after qualifying but, conversely, the vast majority would have carried out regular post-mortem examinations, regardless of whether we moved into farm, equine or companion animal practice. There was a fully functioning post-mortem facility at Hawkshead which did give us the opportunity to observe and take part in such an examination but, oddly to my mind, many were undertaken by pathologists who, for whatever reason, did not want students with them.

We also received some fresh material from local abattoirs, usually condemned viscera with gross evidence of lesions. By definition, however, the vast majority of animals going through abattoirs were healthy and, as a result, the lesions we saw were very minor. These included livers with some evidence of liver fluke damage (thickened bile ducts and the occasional presence of the parasite *Fasciola hepatica),* cattle livers showing telangiectasia (dark spots on the surface caused by small dilated and coalescing blood vessels), and *Muellerius* spp lungworm lesions in the lungs of sheep. None of these posed any real threat to human health but were removed and condemned for aesthetic reasons since they wouldn't look too appetising on the butcher's tray. We received far less practical teaching with companion animal and horse pathology.

Part of our training at that time was supplemented by visits to Luton abattoir, Letchworth bacon factory and a poultry slaughter and package plant to observe the slaughter processes. In particular, we observed the implementation of meat hygiene procedures through inspection and its role in effectively identifying and removing any part of the carcass destined for the food chain that was unsuitable. There was an option to spend longer periods of time at these premises but I never took advantage of this. To be honest, I found all such premises at that time to be very depressing as my interest was in treating, not killing, animals.

Each student had to undergo a period of six months of what was referred to at that time as 'seeing practice' – effectively spending six months of your holiday period in the last three years shadowing and learning from vets predominantly in practice. The requirement is still there today but is now referred to as EMS (extra-mural study) or EMR (extra-mural rotation).

One compulsory placement was to spend time in a government veterinary investigation (VI) centre, where farm animal post-mortem examinations were being undertaken on a daily basis and where we could consider the theory we had learned in the classroom in the context of real 'on farm' problems. My decision to spend two weeks at my local laboratory at Worcester was to have a long-lasting impact on me. It was where my career path took me, working in the VI Service and its subsequent reincarnations for the last 30 years of my career. Each VI centre (and at that time there were 24 located strategically around England and Wales) served the local farming community. They provided a diagnostic service to the surrounding farms through the local veterinary practices, which submitted carcasses for post-mortem examination and samples for laboratory testing.

The Worcester laboratory was in Block C of what was a series of single storey 'temporary' wartime buildings that are still occupied today. During my time at the lab in 1972 there were three veterinary investigation officers (VIO), only two of whom were actually there at the time. I never met the third officer, Don Gibbons, because he was working away on a swine vesicular disease outbreak that was rampant at the time – the first time it had been recorded in the UK. Over the next 10 years, 532 cases involving a total of 322,081 pigs were confirmed before the disease was eradicated from this country in 1982. The laboratory was also staffed by a team of laboratory scientists who undertook the laboratory testing – particularly bacteriology and parasitology – a post-mortem room support worker and an office team.

The senior vet was Ian Shaw, who played a significant role in improving the understanding of border disease in sheep and goats. The second vet was Eddie Winkler, who had previously visited my father's ailing poultry. They were referred to as veterinary investigation officers – and that is exactly what they did – investigate disease outbreaks. These two weeks gave me the opportunity to observe a large number of post-mortem examinations on farm animals and see and recognise the more common pathological presentations. I was fortunate that the post-mortem room attendant was away on holiday during my time at the laboratory and, owing to my enthusiastic approach in the PM room, I was shown how to open up the carcasses and display the viscera for the VIO to examine, assess and sample. I left more convinced that pathology was a fascinating science but did not realise at that time it would prove to be my eventual career choice.

Spending two weeks at a VI centre was compulsory during my time at college and represented a great opportunity for me to gain good practical post-mortem and pathology experience. This is no longer the case as the veterinary schools decided one by one that it should be a voluntary choice. I supervised successive generations of extra-mural students during my time as a VIO and saw a real difference between the often disinterested students who were forced to spend time with us and those who chose to come, the majority of which were keen and gave good feedback on their experiences.

Why was a compulsory VI centre visit removed from the EMS programme? I suspect for a variety of reasons. Firstly, there was a recognition that the profession was changing and, in particular, that the majority of undergraduates would be working in companion animal and not farm practice. No doubt these were my disinterested students. Secondly, and intrinsically linked, the number of VI centres halved between 1972 and 2013, and is set to reduce again. In the same time the number of students has more than doubled, thus creating the logistical problem of finding sufficient placements.

There are currently two veterinary schools, London and Liverpool, that have a VI centre (referred to as a surveillance centre) embedded within the university and a third at Nottingham located next door to the Sutton Bonington laboratory. Students at these colleges get the chance to spend time observing post-mortem examinations in the way that I did and have the chance to carry out such an examination where possible.

I do have a concern that, judging by my observations of successive groups of students I have supervised on EMS, the depth and breadth of the modern veterinary curriculum means the practical teaching of pathology may still be lacking. However, I realise that this will vary from one school to the next. I do genuinely believe, however, that my time at Worcester with Ian Shaw and Eddie Winkler was a pivotal moment in my own career – when pathology as a component part of a disease investigation began to really mean something.

The veterinary course is like building a wall. All the bricks are individually important for the structure of the wall but when they are laid together it has structure and function. Teaching the various disciplines is important but the ability to merge these is what makes a competent veterinary surgeon. In my day, these disciplines were taught completely separate from each other. But recognising the problem this creates, a more modern trend is to attempt to interlink the course components from the outset. This has been referred to as the Nottingham approach, after the new veterinary school in the city that opened in 2006. Its aim was to introduce aspects of surgery, radiology and anaesthesia when anatomy was taught in year one, so not only the discipline but its application and eventual integration is understood at an early stage.

The pathology course during my time as an undergraduate was a very full one and one subject I particularly enjoyed was parasitology. This is divided into two main branches: ectoparasites, the study of parasites living on the host such as lice and fleas, and endoparasites, such as worms, that live inside the body. Parasites are an important cause of health and welfare problems across all species and those of importance are many and varied.

Before moving on to the clinical aspects of diagnosis, treatment and control it is vital to understand the basic life cycles of the more important types and how to recognise the parasite itself, or the eggs or oocysts shed in faeces that we rely on to assess endoparasite burdens.

The life cycles of parasites can be fascinating and complex and we learned many of these in order to pass the parasitology part of the pathology exams. A thorough knowledge of these underpins our ability to develop control strategies. I may be wrong but the modern student does not have these life cycles at their fingertips in the way they were drummed into us in the 1970s. I know this because I have often asked students to explain one to me.

Some life cycles are direct, such as those of the majority of nematode gastro-intestinal worms. The mature worm lives in the gut and lays eggs that are voided in faeces and pass on to the pasture. Depending on ambient temperature and moisture, these eggs hatch to larvae, which in turn pass through a series of developmental stages before they move up the herbage ready to be ingested, swallowed and begin the life cycle over again.

The time taken for larvae to be ingested at one end and for faeces to appear at the other end is referred to as the pre-patent period and for nematode worms this is between 18 and 22 days. Certain worms such as *Haemonchus contortus*, the barber's pole worm, and *Ostertagia* spp can become inhibited in the wall of the fourth stomach (or abomasum), thus extending the normal pre-patent period and life cycle, before literally bursting out in large numbers and causing severe clinical signs. Other parasites such as liver fluke (*Fasciola hepatica*) have an indirect life cycle and this involves an additional host through which the parasite must pass to complete it. In the case of liver fluke, it is the mud snail *Galba truncatula*. The adult liver fluke can be found in the gall bladder and bile ducts of the liver in affected ruminants (mainly sheep and cattle). Mature fluke lay eggs and these pass in the bile directly into the upper small intestine, before being carried down through the gut to be passed in faeces on to the pasture. The eggs hatch into miracidia, which must then find the mud snail, into which they penetrate, going through further developmental stages in the snail itself, before emerging as cercaria. These encyst on the pasture to prevent them drying out before being eaten again by a passing ruminant, in which the life cycle continues.

A thorough knowledge of this fluke life cycle (including its extended eight to 12-week pre-patent period) again gives us the ability to identify potential control points. In this example we can either treat the parasite while in the ruminant using products called flukicides or we can control the snail habitats by fencing and drainage. When I qualified, there were a number of molluscicides that could be sprayed on to wet areas to kill the snails but these have now all been banned.

Our practical sessions in parasitology consisted mainly of undertaking worm or fluke egg counts – literally counting the number of eggs voided per gram of faeces. We did this by shaking measured amounts of faeces with mainly a saturated salt solution, then counting eggs seen down the microscope in a specialised glass counting chamber known as a McMaster slide. Knowing the dilution rates, a simple calculation gave the faecal egg count – a potential measure of the weight of infection present. In companion animal parasitology time was spent looking at skin scrapings and hair plucks for the characteristic morphological appearance of, for example, sarcoptic, chorioptic or demodectic mange mites – each one of which had a particular shape to its body or legs. This was the classic discipline in which the steeplechase spot practical exams were widely used, coupled with written exams testing mainly our knowledge of life cycles.

I often ask myself why I can still remember the Latin (proper) names of less well known parasites, including some of the ectoparasites affecting poultry such as *Cuclotogaster heterographus* and *Menacanthus stramineus,* from 40 years ago, when nowadays I cannot remember what I did two days ago.

I was taught virology at a time when veterinary virology was still very much a developing discipline, with many grey areas in our understanding of even what we consider as common endemic viral diseases today. A prime example is bovine viral diarrhoea (BVD), possibly one of the most important and widely distributed viruses in the UK cattle population. I was taught that the virus causes pyrexia (high temperature), diarrhoea and abortion but can also cause congenital abnormalities such as poor development of the cerebellum. The main diagnostic tool available to us was paired serology – literally taking a blood sample on the first day that infection was suspected, then taking a follow-up sample around two weeks later to see if there had been a rise in BVD antibody between the two samples. This is still a commonly used test.

We were also aware of a further manifestation of this condition referred to as mucosal disease. This is invariably a fatal disease in which affected cattle often grow poorly before a terminal decline in which they develop severe mouth and oesophageal ulceration, with similar damage throughout the gut and a severely compromised immune system. It was to be 10 years after I qualified that Professor Joe Brownlie, an eminent veterinary virologist, discovered the mechanism by which these clinical cases develop. BVD can cross the placenta and invade the foetus/embryo, something that was known during my time at college. Mr Brownlie was able to demonstrate the virus was assimilated into the developing foetus before its own immune system became developed. Once this immune system was active, the BVD virus was not recognised as being a foreign protein. The foetus then continued to grow literally full of virus and was eventually born and referred to as a PI or persistently infected animal that was BVD antibody naïve but virus positive. Clinical mucosal disease itself then developed as a result of a second BVD viral insult or 'super-infection', either due to mutation of the virus already infecting the calf or from another field strain of virus. This may be complicated but it is vital for the modern veterinary surgeon and farm client to understand.

Immunology was in the curriculum but my recollection was we focused very much on the theory of the immune system, at a time when it was still a relatively new science. There has been a massive increase in the range of tests now available for the diagnosis of viral and other diseases as our knowledge of immunology and its application to modern diagnostic techniques has evolved. I remember during my time in practice in the 1970s and early 1980s how long we had to wait for serology and virology test results to return, whereas now we have tests carried out at the animal's pen that are able to give immediate results of great accuracy.

One part of the virology department that remained a mystery to most of us during our course was a high containment isolation unit on the Camden Town site in which most of the RVC virology research was undertaken. We could see the porthole-like windows of this self-contained building with yellow walls as we passed by, which not surprisingly earned it the name Yellow Submarine.

Having been taught animal husbandry and veterinary hygiene as an introductory subject in years one and two, I continued my studies during the middle part of the course as our second BVetMed exams were to be based on pathology and animal husbandry.

We began to focus on animal husbandry in more detail, getting to grips with nutrition, particularly of farm animals. Acronyms, which I have since used throughout my veterinary career, abounded such as ME or metabolisable energy, RDP or rumen degradable protein, and CP or crude protein. We were taught the fundamentals of ration analysis and dietary constituent quality, using in particular a Ministry of Agriculture, Fisheries and Food (MAFF, the forerunner of Defra) booklet titled *Rations for Livestock*. I still have my copy! Other topics covered included animal housing across species and the milking parlour and milking routines (with options to go along to Boltons Park Farm to take part). We also had a number of practical sessions on pasture management, including the field identification of grass and other plants that contribute to good, average and poor pasture.

The animal husbandry project I was allocated was a fairly obscure one and involved poultry. My group was charged with the task of assessing a number of different rations each containing differing dietary constituents which had variable goitrogenic effects on thyroid development. A goitrogen effectively suppresses thyroid gland function, leading to enlargement. The most goitrogenic ration was one containing a high proportion of rapeseed. The project ended with the broilers – birds that grow rapidly and are slaughtered at only a few weeks old – being humanely euthanised and the thyroid glands dissected out and weighed. The broilers on the high rapeseed diet had the largest thyroid glands, confirming the goitrogenic effects of the high rapeseed inclusion. This was a potentially important factor when devising rations for such birds.

After one year and two terms, we sat our second BVetMed exams in the whole subject of pathology and animal husbandry and veterinary hygiene. I was particularly fortunate in my animal husbandry pre-clinical exams because it was a subject I really enjoyed revising. On the day of the exam, however, and for some unknown reason, I awoke very early (maybe 5am) and started going through revision material in my head. I suddenly realised I had missed a chunk of work out completely and, in a bit of a panic, I retrieved the necessary notes covering equine and canine management and read them through. A major part of this was on dog breeding and kennelling. Imagine my surprise when I had the chance to answer two questions from that morning's revision which could not have been any fresher in my mind.

I was one of only two students in the year to gain a distinction in Animal Husbandry and Veterinary Hygiene and I also passed my pathology exams. Next stop, final year!

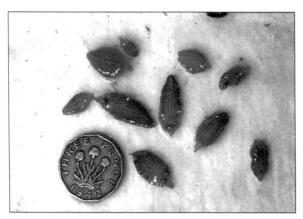

Liver fluke and a pre-decimal threepenny piece – still a
major problem today!

Chapter 7
The Pressure Mounts – Final Exams Approach

Although we began the clinical part of the course at the beginning of our third year, it was not until the second BVetMed exams had taken place that we focused solely on medicine and surgery. One major difference between my final year and that of the modern student was my lectures continued throughout the year, even up to the weeks before final exams. The current curriculum tends to leave the final year lecture-free, focusing (quite correctly in my view) on consolidating the theory via directed learning procedures, workshops, discussion groups and, most importantly, practical hands-on experience.

You can always tell the final year students at vet school – they are the ones with the stethoscope around their necks and are always looked at with envy by the lower years. Although we all enjoyed the year, the spectre of finals was always there in the backs of our minds, coupled with the excitement and apprehension of getting our first jobs.

We began to observe or 'sit in' on consultations with the college medical and surgical staff, and to observe and assist in the operating theatres and with other clinical procedures. Although my major area of interest was in farm work, sadly this was the area least well covered during my final year. The emphasis was heavily biased towards small animals and equine and I am told that is still the case today. Students I have supervised tell me they have received more teaching on canine orthopaedics than they have on sheep and more on cardiology than they have on goats.

It is a fact of life, I suppose, that college teaching staff tend to be specialists and keen on their specific areas of expertise. So if you have world class veterinary orthopaedic surgeons, they will need a large chunk of teaching time to pass on what they consider to be a necessary grounding in their specialism. Conversely, if you lack staff with knowledge and, more importantly enthusiasm, in a subject area, this area may be overlooked. Bringing expertise from outside the college is often undertaken but during financial cutbacks and constraints it is often the external teaching staff who are the first casualties. I know this first-hand as at one stage I provided a half-day on goat health and welfare at all existing vet schools and this invitation is now extended only by three schools. This reduction is not just my poor teaching as I know other external speakers have also not been invited back.

The RVC now has the world-renowned Queen Mother Hospital for Small Animals at Hawkshead. This does undoubtedly provide a high and varied throughput of clinical material, although other colleges have similar facilities. One problem with clinical material going through veterinary colleges is that it is second opinion/referral case material – interesting, complex and thought-provoking but often far removed from the day-to-day clinical load when in practice.

Equally, although I know the importance of working in a profession that does not stand still, I am concerned that the expectations of many of today's new graduates on qualifying may often be diminished by their inability to live up to the ideals instilled in them during the course. What do I mean by this? Simply that much of the caseload they experience in their final years relies on a range of complex procedures such as MRI (magnetic resonance imaging) scans, CT (computerised tomography) scans, electrocardiography and cardiac echograms that the majority of practices will not possess, leading to them having to offer a 'second class' service or to refer.

Similarly, students are shown complex treatment protocols, such as cancer radiotherapy and chemotherapy, and limb prosthetics, all of which are again way out of reach of the average practitioner. There is a degree of disillusionment that often hits students after the euphoria of qualifying, getting a first job and a wage begins to wear off. This can be compounded, particularly in small rural practices, by a feeling of isolation as the direct social interaction with student friends at college becomes replaced by interaction via social networking, which is never the same.

We did not have the toys and gadgets of the modern student. Radiography was the primary diagnostic tool, backed up by laboratory testing and good clinical and differential diagnostic skills. Although many of the small animal cases we experienced at Hawkshead were second opinion cases referred by local practitioners, many were for procedures carried out widely in practice today. The orthopaedic department of the RVC was highly thought of, and it was renowned for its ophthalmic work. Much of this was down to clinicians whose reputations extended beyond the boundaries of the college, such as Lesley Vaughan and Gary

Clayton Jones on the orthopaedic team and Professor Formston (and later Peter Bedford) as ophthalmologists. Many of the small animal cases coming through the hospital were related to spinal problems, and spinal surgery in the known susceptible breeds was a growing specialism at that time.

Another new approach at that time was tibial crest transplant as a procedure for correcting medial patellar luxation in dogs and cats. My hands (as an assistant) also featured in a paper in the *Journal of Small Animal Practice*, holding instruments in an operation to correct 'dry eye', or keratoconjunctivitis sicca, by parotid duct transplant. Peter Bedford had undertaken a series of such operations and was reporting on his findings. As the name suggests, the absence of adequate tear flow across the eye can be serious and this procedure replaces the tears with saliva.

We spent periods of time on rotation at the Beaumont Animals Hospital in Camden Town, which adjoined the Camden Town college site. Most of the animals treated at the college were horses and livestock but some companion animals have always been seen. Records show that during 1828, for example, 16 dogs were admitted.

As the years passed, domestic companion animals became increasingly important in society and the university widened this aspect of its curriculum. Accordingly, it started building the Beaumont Hospital in 1932. The facility was completed and opened in 1933 as an undergraduate teaching hospital. A bequest of £25,000 came from the will of a wealthy Yorkshire woman, Sarah Martin Grove-Grady. She was the daughter of J Beaumont of Huddersfield, who had helped establish the first horse ambulance service in London. The hospital has remained open ever since and, like the Windmill Theatre, even kept working during the Second World War when the rest of the college was evacuated. In 2010, the trustees of the Jean Sainsbury Animal Welfare Trust made a substantial one-off donation towards the complete refurbishment of the hospital. Now renamed the Beaumont Sainsbury Animal Hospital, it currently offers RVC final year students the opportunity to work and gain experience in a busy city centre practice.

In addition to spending time gaining experience at the Beaumont Hospital, it also provided the first case in my final year casebook, which provided a summary of cases we experienced during extra-mural studies mainly undertaken away from the college. My girlfriend Diane's family dog, a Scottie cross called Rufty, developed a swelling under his tongue, which was rapidly increasing in size. I had never seen anything like it before but thought it may have been either a grass seed or splinter that had become embedded under the tongue or possibly a salivary cyst. Diane and I took Rufty to the Beaumont's clinic as members of the public and luckily we were seen by one of the housemen, a recently qualified vet whom I knew quite well. His view was that it was almost certainly a salivary swelling, referred to as a ranula. A ranula (also referred to as a mucocele), results from rupture of the duct carrying saliva from a local salivary gland to the duct where it opens into the mouth. In Rufty's case, as the swelling was under the tongue, it was the sub-mandibular salivary gland on the same side that was the source of the increasing swelling. It was arranged for the offending salivary gland to be removed and I was able to assist, hence the case's inclusion in my book. One major difference between my casebook and one of today's students' was the distinct lack of photographs. I drew diagrams to explain the association between the swelling, the duct and the sub-mandibular gland. Now, modern digital images can be readily taken, reviewed and printed for case inclusion.

On reflection, I received good background practical advice on the small animal side, both at college and also in my EMS placements. I also received some excellent training in equine medicine and surgery at college, although as a matter of choice I did spend less time on this during my placements.

The majority of equine case submissions during my time at the RVC were second opinion, having been referred by veterinary surgeons from far and wide. They seemed to fall into three main categories, namely lameness, colic and tooth problems, together with some stable 'vices' that could be controlled by surgery.

On rotation within this department, we had the chance to meet the owners of the referral cases and take a history prior to carrying out our clinical examination. As many of the lameness cases were accompanied by their owner or stable staff, many of whom were young and female, my male-only student group enjoyed putting not only the horse but also its attendant through their paces. When assessing lameness in a horse, it is usually best to observe the animal trotting away from you and back towards and past you. We had a phrase said quietly between us that 'we must watch the horse this time'.

Most of the clinical examinations were undertaken without the array of ancillary aids available to the modern equine specialist, who has both ultrasound and complex computer-generated X-ray imagery at his or her disposal. We relied on the skill of the college equine staff, who often used nerve blocks to de-sensitise specific areas of the foot so they could locate the site of damage. Many referred cases were either related to navicular disease, associated with degenerative change to the navicular bone within the hoof, or to chronic laminitis, a specific problem often seen in aged horses or over-fat ponies. One golden piece of advice I was given by Lesley Vaughan was to watch the head of the horse. As the painful foot hits the ground, the horse will drop its head due to the discomfort. This advice was accompanied by his experience of watching ponies and donkeys pulling carts on his Mediterranean travels. He found it much easier to gauge head movement if the affected animal wore a hat and many such animals will wear a straw hat to keep the sun out of their eyes. We never suggested that our equine patients should be given a hat to wear during our examination but this advice has stuck with me throughout my career. It applies not only to horses but also to lame cows – a species with which I had much more involvement.

Equine colic cases were always a big draw for us as they invariably resulted in often heroic surgery in our attempts to save them. Colic in horses is a generic term applied to severe abdominal pain that results from gas build-up in the intestinal tract, which in turn may be due to blockages or twists and torsions of the gut itself. Affected horses were often driven to the college for assessment and treatment and, as these are true emergencies, they turned up at any time of the day or night.

The animals were initially assessed by taking their pulse, temperature and heart rate to gauge the severity of their pain. Auscultation of the abdomen by stethoscope gave us some idea of whether the pain was due to gas build-up under pressure or whether a blockage had caused total stasis of the bowel. Rectal examination could then be used to literally feel the lengths of affected gut through the relatively thin rectal wall. Many cases with blockages were managed medically, most frequently by the administration of large amounts of liquid paraffin by stomach tube, a skill we all learned at this time.

It was the surgical cases that provided the most excitement, with any opportunity for an assistant role always very popular and sought after. Horses are large and neither anaesthesia nor surgery of the abdomen are easy options, particularly if the animal is shocked and in pain. The afflicted animals were anaesthetised by intravenous injection in a padded box to protect them if they fell awkwardly during anaesthesia induction or when they were returned to the box to recover. After they 'dropped' they were winched up by a small mobile crane and gantry that moved them to the operating table, where they were intubated and attached to a gaseous anaesthetic machine to maintain anaesthesia. Surgery was often spectacular, as length after length of gut came out through the incision and was deflated to allow gas or ingesta to escape. Our role was either to monitor depth of anaesthesia, with patients often at high risk due to the shock and pressure on the diaphragm, or to assist the surgeon, including stitching up at the end of the operation. We then had to monitor recovery back in the padded box and continue to check daily during hospitalisation and recovery, administering antibiotic or pain relief under supervision.

Many of the equine patients were hospitalised out at Hawkshead and were monitored by the duty student group on rotation. One weekend when I was on duty, I took Diane out with me to show her what I did. She was moving from box to box patting and talking to the horses in turn when I suddenly heard her shriek. I rushed to see what was wrong, only to find her staring ashen-faced at the side of a horse's face she had just been idly patting that had a large hole where a molar tooth had recently been extracted, and that we were irrigating daily.

Equine dentistry is not for the faint-hearted because the molar teeth are very long as they continue to grow during the horse's life and are deeply embedded in the jaw and maxilla. The approach used on this horse was, under general anaesthesia, to loosen the tooth in the mouth along its gum margins and to then cut the skin on the outer surface of the face immediately above the root of the tooth. Using a trephine, we then drilled a hole down to the tooth root and, using a chisel and mallet, hammered the tooth out into the mouth. The incision was then left open, as Diane discovered, for us to irrigate daily, with the opening slowly closing over. Today, almost all abscessed teeth can be removed from within the mouth using the proper tools and new techniques. The method I experienced left permanent scars and disfigurement, so is rarely used now.

As a student, you most often learn by exposure to and interaction with dedicated staff who share their experiences and skills with you. You can also learn from your own mistakes, and those of others, and it was the latter that became the talk of the year. The unfortunate 'other' in the instance I'm going to describe was a young and fairly recently qualified veterinary surgeon who was working in the equine surgery department. The case I was assigned to was a horse admitted to the college as a second opinion case, having developed a condition referred to as 'crib-biting'. This is an abnormal, compulsive behaviour or stereotypy seen in some horses and considered a stable vice. It involves the horse grabbing a solid object, such as the stable door or fence rail, with its incisors, then arching its neck, pulling against the object, and sucking in air. Windsucking is a related behaviour whereby the horse arches its neck and sucks air into the windpipe without needing to grab a solid object. The condition can have serious consequences, leading to weight loss and predisposing the animal to both colic and stomach ulcers. It can also in time lead to abnormal tooth wear. The behaviour can also affect an animal's potential value, discouraging potential purchasers. There have been considerable advances in our understanding of this condition from the time that I dealt with our referred case. At the time, it was referred to simply as a vice resulting from boredom or stress since the condition invariably began while the horse was stabled, not at grass. It was also considered to be a learned vice, meaning horses copied each other.

Our case was scheduled for a surgery involving Forssell's procedure, in which the muscles of the underside of the neck are exposed and either cut or removed with a view to preventing the mechanical process leading to the vice itself, i.e.

the horse is physically unable to grasp the solid structure with its mouth. It was a particularly invasive type of surgery, often with a degree of success but not without its problems, primarily associated with local wound breakdown.

Our case went well initially. Anaesthesia was uneventful and the horse was on the operating table on its back with its neck outstretched and ready for surgery. We discussed the anatomy of the area, palpated the muscles due to be exposed and the house surgeon made the initial incision. We then began to identify each muscle in turn, separating and exposing each one. Suddenly, there was a very fine spray of blood being released under pressure which gradually increased in intensity until we were all being showered. During the separation of the muscles the carotid artery had been incised. This vessel carries blood under pressure to the head structures, running up the neck under the very muscles we were examining. Our surgeon let out a scream and, for a reason I've never been able to fathom, began to sing at the top of his voice, presumably in panic. Luckily, a more senior member of the surgical team was on hand to assist, the bleeding was eventually stopped and the operation completed. My lesson was to consider *every* possible anatomical structure that could be damaged or at risk during surgery, not simply the target organ or structure.

There have been many modifications of the Forssell's procedure, some of which are still carried out. These involve cutting the nerve supply (neurectomy) to the muscle and not removing the muscle itself, as well as other modifications involving micro-surgery by laser.

One particular individual in the equine department who I remember fondly was Dr Greatorex. This is partly for his patient equine medicine teaching but more particularly for his enthusiastic teaching on poisonous plants and their potential effects on livestock. I had an interest in plants as a boy, when I collected and pressed wild flowers, and I really took to this topic. We had lectures on the subject but my lasting memory was of the practical sessions that took place in the post-mortem room at Hawkshead.

Dr Greatorex had spent time gathering specimens of the more common, and some unusual, plants, shrubs and trees that could potentially be harmful to grazing livestock. Laid out on the tables were branches from yew, oak, laurel and laburnum, alongside plants such as St John's wort, ragwort and hemlock, with tubers from plants such as water dropwort. I qualified with a very deep knowledge of these plants, including their proper names. For example, yew is *Taxus baccata*, oak is *Quercus robu* and ragwort is *Senecio jacobaea*. It is knowledge that I retain 40 years on.

Poisonous plant teaching in modern veterinary schools is a far cry from the grounding I received at the RVC. I found this out when I ran a seminar for final year students at my old college 35 years after I qualified. One question I asked the students to consider concerned the sudden deaths of a number of cattle on the edge of some woodland and to consider likely causes. One such cause was poisonous plants, shrubs or trees. Without exception, each group struggled to come up with any correct answers and more than half resorted to searching the internet and presenting me with a list of plants, many of which we never see in the UK.

Although my ambition from day one was to be a farm animal vet, it was the farm part of the final year course that I found the most disappointing. Although the clinical notes were sound, it was the lack of any real farm animal cases coming through the vet schools that was most frustrating. The arrival of even a calf with diarrhoea was enough to get the word spreading through the final year, as we all clambered to see it and get involved. I suppose with hindsight, the RVC being sited on the outskirts of London and away from the main farming areas should have made the reason for this shortage of cases obvious. Most of the cases that were referred were from local practices, either as second opinion cases where help or specialist treatment was required, such as a valuable calf being placed on a drip. Some cases were also purchased from local farms purely for teaching purposes. They all gave us the chance to practise our diagnostic skills, including taking blood samples, giving injections, passing a stomach tube and so on. We could follow most cases through to conclusion, and that may have been euthanasia, another opportunity to learn this procedure, and post-mortem examination.

All modern veterinary schools recognised the need to have a regular throughput of clinical material and regular contact by students with clinical cases. In slightly differing ways, each college now either has its own large animal practice, providing a service to local livestock keepers in the way any conventional practice would, or has a close relationship with a neighbouring practice. In both situations, students are able to accompany the qualified vet out on his or her round and to become intimately involved in any case material presented or in routine procedures such as foot trimming cows and pregnancy testing. During my time there the RVC did not have this facility. Nevertheless, my enthusiasm was not dampened and the majority of my practical experience was gained during my EMS studies.

During the final year, we were encouraged to carry out a mini project. This could be in any area of veterinary work but there were a few specific projects up for grabs and a group of four of us opted for one assessing the incidence of gastric ulceration in pigs at slaughter.

The pig has a similar gut to humans, including a single stomach, and occasionally develops ulcers in the lining. In severe cases, these ulcers can kill a pig if it perforates and releases gastric juices into the abdominal cavity, resulting in peritonitis. Most cases are not obvious until the pig is killed and the stomach examined.

At the time of our survey, there was a strong feeling these ulcers could be widespread and having a harmful effect on pig growth rates, and hence productivity, thus taking the animal longer to reach slaughter weight and eating more as a result. The exact cause was not known, although some believed it could be related to food particle size. We received 30 to 40 pig stomachs from a local abattoir every Wednesday. Our task was to open each one, tip the food into a bowl and weigh the amount of feed present. We had to grade the fineness of the feed particles and then examine the actual inner surface of the stomach wall.

Ulcers in pigs develop around an area referred to as the *pars oesophagea,* which is on the stomach wall where the oesophagus enters at the cardia, and which has the same keratinised lining as the oesophagus, making it a very obvious structure. Having identified an ulcer, we then had to assess whether there was one or more, measure the diameter and depth, and draw them on to a pro-forma diagram. Our work formed the basis of a paper published several years later in the *Veterinary Record.*

EMS was a compulsory and vital part of our teaching, and still is. It recognises that students are unable to gain the experiences of day-to-day veterinary life and its routine in the relative ivory tower in which the bulk of the teaching takes place. The stipulation has not changed; essentially all veterinary undergraduates have to spend 26 weeks of their holiday period during the clinical years gaining veterinary experience outside college. Most of this time is spent at veterinary practices in a phase often referred to as 'seeing practice'. During my EMS, I spent most of my time at the practice of Renfrew and Sons in Broadway, a small village on the edge of the Cotswolds. I also spent more time at the practice in Evesham where I had helped out in my pre-college years. I also spent two weeks at Beaumont Hospital in Camden Town, which was useful as I could stay with Diane, who lived just around the corner. My final two weeks were spent at the Worcester Veterinary Investigation Centre, described earlier.

I had no problem in finding a placement near my home, which at least kept my costs down. Today's students find it more difficult, particularly in gaining farm animal experience, and there are three main reasons for this.

Firstly, the student numbers have increased dramatically, from fewer than 300 qualifying each year to more than 700 students in their final year today, and these numbers continue to increase.

Secondly, and I'm referring specifically here to farm animal and true mixed practices, the number of available practices for this increasing student pool is decreasing almost exponentially. Many true mixed practices are no longer undertaking farm work and have become companion-animal-only concerns. Farms have been getting bigger and fewer, particularly in the dairy sector. These fewer, larger farms require fewer practices to service their veterinary requirements and the demand has also been for more specialist veterinary input. As a result, the farm animal veterinary work tends in smaller mixed practices to be undertaken by only one vet, and this person is usually an older, more senior male. At weekends and when this vet is on holiday, cover is provided by others in the practice, but they undertake little farm animal work routinely and provide emergency cover only. Dissatisfied farms will move to larger, more specialised, farm animal practices, while loyal farm clients will stick with the same practice and their trusted senior experienced vet. When this vet retires, however, other vets in the practice do not have the experience and, more importantly, the competence and confidence to take on the work. The practice then decides to move out of farm work, and the more specialist farm practice picks up the new clients and continues to increase in size. This pattern has been no more apparent than in south-east England, where I worked for the last 19 years of my career. There, I watched the number of practices doing farm work more than halve during that time.

Thirdly, EMS can be expensive. Some travel expenses can be claimed but gaining experience near home or with a relative or friend is on every student's wish list and this in itself will invariably reduce the choice of practices to attend.

To get around these problems, there have been moves over the past few years for final year students to undertake some EMS during term time, when there is less competition for places. Most colleges also now have their own practice or a close liaison with a neighbouring one, giving students year-round access. It is also clear from the EMS students I have supervised that the aims and objectives of the placement, together with specific learning objectives, are made clear to the host practice. This did not seem to be the case when I did my EMS, and although I had the opportunity to observe a wide range of clinical cases, the opportunity to actually participate was minimal. From discussion with fellow students in my year, this situation was not unique to me. Today's practices take their obligations as teachers of EMS students far more seriously; quite a few of us got the feeling that we were being granted a huge favour by being allowed to spend time with them. This seems very ungrateful of me but, as ever, hindsight is a wonderful way of assessing an experience. I just wish I had been given the opportunities during my EMS placements that many of today's students have.

As an example, rectal examination was, and still is, an everyday procedure in dairy cattle work. Its two main functions are either to assess whether or not a cow is pregnant after service (usually by artificial insemination) or to assess any factors that may have made the cow infertile if she has not been on heat, and hence not served. It is a technique we all have to learn and, after donning an arm-length polythene glove, the hand and arm is lubricated ready for insertion into the cow's anus. With your arm inside the cow, you can palpate the cervix, vagina and uterus and also carry out a detailed examination of the ovaries, literally using your fingers and thumb. As the procedure is such a common one to undertake, and as there were 65 of us and only a small number of cows at Hawkshead for us to learn on, it was during our EMS that we were expected to become more skilled.

My problem was that both vets in my main EMS practice were reluctant to let me carry out the procedure, either because they were in a hurry and feared I would slow them down, or because they were concerned the owner of the cows wouldn't like a student interfering with them. I did get the chance to do some rectals but I spent much of my time watching as the vet described what he was doing with phrases such as 'this cow has a large cyst in its right ovary', or 'this cow is pregnant, I can feel some good membrane development'. This lack of real experience was a disadvantage to me in my first practice post.

Today's students are given a much more focused practical grounding, which is enhanced by having lecture-free final years in which the skills learned in the classroom can be put into practice. I did become very skilled at rectal procedures, and even with time became ambidextrous (particularly useful on cold mornings with bare arms), but was essentially right-handed, or more correctly right-armed. Another major change has been the increased use of ultrasound techniques for pregnancy diagnosis and fertility investigation, with the one major advantage that an image of the uterus and its contents can be displayed on a small screen alongside the cow, a clear advance on teaching by imagination as I had experienced.

I spent the remainder of my time observing day-to-day life in two busy rural practices, spending time on the farms, and in the consulting room and operating theatre. I built up my casebook, handed it in and finally completed my 26 weeks EMS. The next step was finals.

Diane and I decided to get married during my final year in 1973. Maybe we were both too young, but we got our parents' blessings and tied the knot on 8 September. I was due to sit my finals in March 1974. We decided to get married at my village church in Church Lench rather than in Diane's parish of Camden Town. We invited many of our respective friends and hired a coach to bring them to what was, in village terms, a big wedding with 'all those folks from London'. After a short honeymoon in Pembrokeshire, I had to return to college and revision. We decided to rent a small flat in a house in Bedford Avenue, High Barnet, with six other girls. At that time, this was an unusual arrangement as flat-sharing was invariably an all-male or all-female affair. To be surrounded by young and very sociable females at a time when the miniskirt was very much in fashion could have been distracting but my newly married status and my determination to do well in my exams kept me focused.

I did find out retrospectively that my parents were concerned that I had made a mistake and that my studies would suffer. But in fact it was just the opposite. Married life in this very happy and relaxed environment away from the college was really conducive to focused study. Diane was brilliant. She was supportive and not at all critical of the hours I had to spend with my nose in my books. My housemates could have been disruptive and noisy but they were not. I was away from the remainder of my year, most of whom were now living in Northumberland Hall, a hall of residence on the Hawkshead campus. I found out each day how stressful life was becoming on the campus as more and more time was spent in the common room discussing revision topics and potentially worrying each other into a disorganised revision schedule. I could remain totally focused without my fellow students and the inevitable distractions of living alongside each other.

Finals eventually arrived and at that time consisted of eight, three-hour examinations extending from Monday through to Thursday night. We then had Friday and the weekend off, before heading into the second week of practicals and oral examinations or vivas. Today's students have it much easier by comparison, with only two or three written papers in their finals. They also have a much fairer and less stressful build-up to these exams, which are supplemented by continual assessment throughout the year. I came through this first week in a haze, it never occurring to me that I knew enough about veterinary medicine and surgery to keep writing for 24 hours. The second week was slightly less stressful but I did get some serious grilling in my vivas, as we all did.

I do have one recollection that I look back on fondly which involved a now very eminent veterinary surgeon, who at that time was a houseman at the college in the department of obstetrics. We were sitting discussing the day's exams when he joined us and I finished up talking one-to-one with him on the way back to the car park. He asked me if I was looking forward to the obstetrics practicals the following day and, slightly tongue in cheek, I said that I was quietly confident but hoped I wouldn't be asked to carry out a pregnancy assessment of a mare (same procedure as cows, by carrying out a rectal examination). I subsequently walked into the obstetrics department for my practical examination, only to be met by the same houseman I had been talking to the night before. To my horror, his first words were: 'Good morning Mr Harwood, I would first like you to examine the mare held in the stocks (a small race into which a horse is placed for detailed examination) and tell me if you think she is pregnant'. My heart sank, thinking I had loaded a gun the night before for him to shoot me down. I donned my gloves with a sinking heart, placed some lubricant on my hand, cupped my fingers as taught and gently inserted my hand into the mare's anus. A broad smile quickly replaced my worried frown – this mare was not only pregnant but I could practically shake hands with the foal and pat it on its head. The mare was due to give birth very shortly to a full-term foal.

Eventually, the day came when final results were to be announced. I still recall us all wandering up and down the corridor at Camden Town, waiting for the notice to go up. My name was there: I had passed my finals. Those of us who had qualified congratulated each other but sadly some of my year did not pass and had to face the spectre of repeating those exams again. All we could do was console and reassure them. I had to wait until I saw Diane later in the day to tell her the news that I was now a veterinary surgeon and Bachelor of Veterinary Medicine.

Shortly afterwards, all successful candidates were sworn in as members of the Royal College of Veterinary Surgeons (RCVS), effectively the profession's governing body, membership of which is a prerequisite to practise the art and skill of veterinary medicine in the UK. Both my mother and father came down to the ceremony held in the great hall in Camden Town when, in alphabetical order, we walked up to the RCVS president, shook his hand and received our scroll of membership. We then stood together, were admitted as members of the RCVS and declared our oath. This has changed slightly from my admission in 1974, and currently goes as follows:

'I promise and solemnly declare that I will pursue the work of my profession with integrity and accept my responsibilities to the public, my clients, the profession and the Royal College of Veterinary Surgeons, and that, above all, my constant endeavour will be to ensure the health and welfare of animals committed to my care.'

The accompanying list showed 46 course members were admitted that day out of the original 65 who started. Along the way, some of our group left the course for varying reasons and a small group had to re-sit finals and qualified later that year. Only one of my year qualified with honours, having gained a distinction in each of the four main subject areas. I qualified as the only other member of my year to gain a distinction in animal husbandry and veterinary hygiene, while three students gained distinctions in veterinary surgery.

Looking back at that list 40 years on, two members of my year have been elected as president of the RCVS, Peter Jinman and Jeremy Davies. Peter was also president of the British Veterinary Association (BVA). Steve Dean is currently chairman of the Kennel Club and was formerly chief executive of the Veterinary Medicines Directorate. I eventually became president of the British Cattle

Veterinary Association and chairman of the Goat Veterinary Society (GVS). My final year colleagues have moved into many diverse areas of work. Some are specialist referral companion animal surgeons, some are highly respected equine vets, others have moved into veterinary research or animal behaviour, while the majority have carved out successful careers as general practitioners.

I know that my parents thoroughly enjoyed their visit to the college to watch my swearing of oath and entry on to the RCVS register, and were both very proud of my achievements. What I did not do, however, and in retrospect it was a mistake, was to attend my university degree presentation ceremony for the University of London. I have attended the graduation ceremonies of my daughters and stepdaughters and recognise the pride one feels when they wear the traditional cap and gown and one joins in the applause as they receive their degree.

We qualified in March, having studied for four years and two terms, whereas the remainder of the university degrees lasted three years and finished in June. We were all working when the graduation days were announced and, as a result, very few of us attended, electing instead to receive our degree through the post. My ceremony would have been held at the Royal Albert Hall, with the degree scroll presented by the chancellor of London University, the Queen Mother. I know in retrospect my parents were disappointed and I do not have a photograph in cap and gown as I never wore one. At the time it was not considered to be such a big event, although perhaps in retrospect it would have been nice to have a photo of me in cap and gown alongside those of my daughters and stepdaughters.

It was a tradition at the RVC, and also I believe at other veterinary colleges within the UK, for the final year to hold a review. This review gave students the chance to let their hair down, use their imaginative skills, poke fun at members of staff and, in our case, raise money for a local charity. Our audience was drawn predominantly from the college, including members of staff who were prepared to be the butt of many of the jokes and sketches, other students and a scattering of people who lived in the locality.

We decided to use as a title the somewhat unimaginative Squitty Squitty, Bang Bang – a Faecal Fantasia, starring Needsum Andrews and Dick van Shyte. It was also referred to as 'A Mike O'Bak – Terry M Johnei Production' heavily based on the name of the bacterium that causes Johne's disease in cattle, *Mycobacterium johnei*. Looking at the programme, it consisted of a series of sketches and mimes involving everyone in the year. In 1974 there were no repercussions after having an opening sketch entitled Miss Gay Britain, starring in no particular order Clive, Stuart, Wink, Thias, Robin, Mike, Chas and Dave. I was cast as a newsreader with Brian and we sat behind a desk reading some 'amusing' latest news items, basing our delivery on the popular TV series *The Two Ronnies*. We got some laughs from the jokey news items we told but received the biggest of all when we stood up from behind the desk in part one, with each of us wearing a jacket and tie visible over the desk, but revealing suspenders, stockings and high heels when we walked off. In the second half, we read the news with very manly voices and then at the end reached down, picked up our handbags and walked off arm-in-arm as if we were going on a date (we could get away with this in 1974). With further childish humour, there was a footnote on the programme that read 'Will the audience please evacuate their stools at the end of the performance'.

I'm sure this type of show still goes on but YouTube has created yet another outlet that students are using today. The RVC has several videos posted featuring both staff and students depicting anything from a spoof job interview to students carrying out imaginary rectal examinations while singing relevant rap songs. Students will never change and each generation thinks it has come up with something different and innovative. The truth is, the majority of it has been done before, albeit via different media.

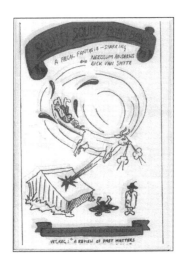

Squitty squitty bang bang, the programme from our final year review!

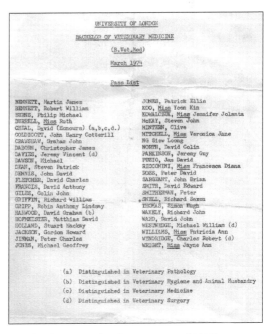

The final year pass list from my year of 1974.

Chapter 8
A Vet at Last – but Stress Levels Rise Again!

We had all been looking at the back of the *Veterinary Record* for our ideal job, as it was there that practices placed their adverts. With a smaller number of us qualifying back in 1974, and with London finishing in March when other college's courses ended a term later, we did have the pick of the jobs, and all of us almost without exception began in our first position shortly after qualifying.

My first job was as a locum for Renfrew and Sons, where I had spent much of my time as a student on EMS. It was only for about two weeks, but gave me the opportunity to see just what it was like to work as a fully qualified vet, without others around to help me and share their wisdom.

I spent much of my time in these weeks helping the practice catch up with some routine tasks, such as castrating calves, disbudding calves and dehorning older cattle, and visiting farms to vaccinate cattle against brucellosis (or contagious abortion in cattle) using an S19 or 45/20 vaccine. These latter vaccines played a major role in eradicating brucellosis and the UK now is officially free of this terrible disease that drove many cattle units out of business. It was also 'zoonotic', essentially a disease of animals that could be picked up by humans. Many vets became infected, mainly from calving infected cows or removing the afterbirth or placenta of an infected cow, because at that time many of them did not wear the arm-length polythene gloves used today. As an aside, I also became infected with brucellosis, but as a student. I inadvertently stuck a needle in my thumb while vaccinating a calf with S19 live brucella vaccine and for many years afterwards I had bouts of flu-like symptoms and fever, hence its name in humans: undulant fever.

These routine procedures seemed to go well and I was beginning to get some confidence as a newly qualified vet. But things took a turn when I was asked to spay a bitch by the principal of the practice, who would be around if I had any problems. The anaesthetic at that time was pentobarbitone by injection. The practice did not possess a gas machine, although the animals were intubated to keep the airways open. The disadvantage was that they took three to four hours to recover fully from the anaesthetic and often had to be kept in overnight if they were operated on late in the day. On occasion, dogs in recovery would go through an excitable phase, often howling uncontrollably. Compare this with modern anaesthesia, with rapid induction agents and anaesthetic maintenance on gas. As a result, recovery is now rapid and trouble free.

I injected the anaesthetic into the foreleg, delivering a measured amount based on the dog's weight, and this worked well. I made the first incision into the abdomen and quickly located the first uterine horn. I applied some gentle pressure and the broad ligament tore, as it should. The ovary appeared, I clamped it off, placed a ligature around the vessels and then incised above my ligature. It held with no bleeding.

I then repeated the procedure on the other horn but on this occasion, after I removed the ovary and second horn, blood began to appear. My ligature had not held and the stump was bleeding. I called for the senior vet and he very calmly helped me locate the stump, re-sutured and the bleeding stopped. I then just had to repeat this procedure on the cervical stump and the complete uterus and both ovaries could be removed. Finally, the abdominal wound needed suturing, the initial layers with cat gut, then single nylon sutures in the skin. I was proud of my stitching. From the outside, it looked neat, with no signs of the problems I had experienced, and the dog went home. As it was almost my last day in the practice, I did not find out until later that this dog took offence at my stiches and licked and chewed some of them out, leaving the incision opening up and gaping. It just so happened that Peter, a fellow newly qualified vet from my year, had just started working full-time in the same practice and he finished up re-stitching my first surgical case.

Diane had accepted the offer of a place at Lanchester Polytechnic in Coventry to undertake her foundation year in the faculty of art and design. She was a talented artist, designer and dressmaker and hoped to begin a full fashion course after completing this initial year. It was imperative, therefore, that I got a job in the vicinity, so in addition to looking through the advertisements in the *Veterinary Record*, I also wrote to a number of practices in the Midlands hoping that one of them might have an upcoming vacancy. I received a reply from EM Pittaway in Coventry, which invited me in for an impromptu interview, before offering me a post as junior assistant. The practice was a very mixed one, dealing with mainly small animals but with a small farm animal side that included some quite large dairy farms and horse clients. It also provided veterinary input to part of the

Royal Agricultural Society showground site at Stoneleigh, provided veterinary cover at Leicester greyhound stadium, and had its own commercial laboratory, LabPak. It sounded like an excellent opportunity to get some experience in a mixed practice environment but I never thought I would have such a varied and often quite stressful time.

In 1974, the usual deal for newly qualified vets was to receive a salary, plus a practice house and car. My car was a second-hand white Austin 1300 and I was to have three accidents in it during my first eight months. On each occasion I ran into the back of another car, usually when I was in a hurry to get to a call or to surgery and was driving too close. Every call to a newly qualified vet is an emergency. Our new house was a large detached bungalow in Tile Hill Lane, the front two rooms of which doubled as a surgery and waiting room. This busy practice had a total of one main surgery in Regent Street and six branch surgeries in Balsall Common and Kenilworth, plus city centre sites in Binley Road, Barker Butts Lane, Foleshill Road and at our bungalow.

The house itself was set back from the road and had a large enclosed back garden. It was unfurnished and as we had little or no money when we moved in, we had to prioritise on what we could afford. We bought a bed, a pine kitchen table and two benches, and two orange tubular steel chairs and cushions, all from Habitat on hire purchase. We were lucky in that we had received many of the day-to-day kitchen items as wedding presents, and there was at least a cooker we could use. Diane bought material and quickly used her sewing skills to make some curtains. We needed a television and bought one in a second-hand shop in Coventry. This sat on an upturned plum box in the corner of the room. We had simple needs at that stage and circumstances forced us to live within our means. Credit cards were not widely available, so the chance of us running up huge debts buying better quality goods that we could not afford was simply not an option. Easily available credit and bank loans make it very easy for young couples now to live the lifestyle they want, without having to work and save for it in advance.

We also had a large garden, much to my dad's delight. He came over from Evesham with my mother and helped us knock it into shape as it had become quite overgrown. There was a large globe artichoke at the end of the garden and lawns near the house. We turned the area in-between into a vegetable garden. It also had a large and very productive grapevine growing in the conservatory attached to the house. Not bad for a first real house and an instant magnet for Diane's newly found college friends.

Over the past few years, I have been tutoring on new graduate training courses mainly for the British Cattle Veterinary Association (BCVA), and have had regular discussions about how traumatic it can be for young people when they get their first job and move away from the 'comfort blanket' that is college life. Graduates also suddenly find themselves on their own and away from student friends, maybe in a small isolated town or village. Being married helped in that respect as at least I had someone to come home to each evening. Life is now much easier from a social perspective for new graduates. They have Facebook and other social media sites so they can regularly keep in touch with each other and share their successes and failures.

We had nothing like this and in a very short time I lost touch with most of my year colleagues and friends. What these training courses have underlined is that I did not receive the help and support I needed, and all new graduates continue to need, when I started full-time work in Coventry. This was due mainly to the heavy and continuous workload immediately imposed on vets, which meant I had quickly to get up to speed and play my part. The best practices now recognise the importance of easing their new graduates in gently, giving one-to-one guidance and support, introducing them to farm clients, debriefing when problems are identified, and, perhaps most importantly, being available instantly via mobile phones, a useful item we did not have. I know in retrospect I took quite a few knocks during my time in Coventry, specifically in small animal surgery, which I quickly began to avoid if I could.

I was put rapidly on the daily rota of morning, afternoon and evening surgeries at the many locations around the city and surrounding towns and villages. I was also given the responsibility of looking after the local RSPCA kennels. I had one day when I was the lead vet for routine surgical operations. I also began to undertake some farm visits and, in time, Greyhound stadium duties. Oddly enough, I was never given the evening surgery at my bungalow and this was covered by one of the other vets. At the start, I did have one week in which I sat in on consultations by the principal at the main Regent Street surgery but after that I was on my own. I was given the Binley Road surgery as my regular base – on the other side of Coventry from where I lived – and surgery was held there twice daily at 8.30am and 6pm. As there were so many surgeries to cover, with only five vets in total and with each of us having a half-day off every week, there was some inevitable shuffling of surgery rotas, and within a short time I had visited them all.

My nightmare day each week was Wednesday, specifically the afternoon and evening. I began with the Balsall Common surgery. This ran from 4.30pm until 5pm and was usually fairly quiet. I then had to move to the Kenilworth surgery, which ran from 5pm until 5.30pm, and this was around five miles from Balsall Common, so I was always late arriving. Luckily, this surgery was also fairly quiet but I was often not there until 5.15pm and, as a new graduate, I was invariably slow and overran.

The next step was my real weekly nightmare because I then had to drive over to my own surgery in Binley Road, the second busiest in the practice, open (at least in theory) between 6pm and 7pm. This was six miles away and I had to travel during rush hour. I was always late and could never park as the car park was full, so I finished up leaving my car in the street around the corner. I still remember vividly that sinking feeling when I saw the waiting room full of people and their pets waiting to see me. I would often not finish until 8pm or even later. Most modern practices now operate an appointment system, which does make it much easier to plan your days and evenings, and is much preferred by clients. If I was also on night duty on Wednesday I often had to rush off to a calving, leaving a bewildered group of owners waiting for another vet to finish their own surgery and come and take over. It was a fairly chaotic time but I did begin to develop a routine and, more importantly, began to work more quickly.

Every branch surgery had a receptionist who opened up in the morning, met the pet owners and generally looked after the building and the attending vet. In my case, and particularly on Wednesday evening, they had to cover for me as I was almost always late. I was fortunate at Binley Road to have a really excellent receptionist called Joan, who was what I term a 'people person'. She lived locally and seemed to know an extraordinary number of the owners who turned up. Joan also had an uncanny way of remembering pets, their names and even family members. She was a fantastic asset to me and gave me tremendous support and encouragement.

Joan's other quite remarkable skill was animal handling. This is something that can be learned but many of the best handlers, particularly farm stockpeople, seem to have an inbuilt ability which seems to instil confidence in the animals themselves. She was one such person. Most of the time, it was simply that Joan held a dog firmly while I gave it an injection, or held a cat while I took its temperature. The firm, yet confident, grip meant the animal rarely struggled. What I did notice, however, was if a gentle grip was not enough to control the unwanted movements, it would tighten but the patter would remain unchanged. Joan would say: 'There's a good dog, you're such a good dog aren't you', and at the same pitch and intensity while the owners would continue to look on in admiration. Some dogs never gave up but neither did my trusty receptionist and her grip tightened even more. On occasion, I watched the dog or cat begin to go blue and the eyes roll, but the grip never wavered and neither did the banter. No owner ever complained and neither did I. Every surgery should have such a receptionist.

It was at Binley Road that I met a number of real characters. One such woman could be seen regularly pulling her shopping trolley and I had noticed her a few times before I spotted her in the waiting room. Joan gave me the background. 'She is a bit eccentric. She lives just around the corner and has a passion for tortoises. She even takes the tortoises for walks in her shopping trolley'.

Sure enough, in she came with two tortoises. One had badly discharging eyes, which I bathed and prescribed some eye ointment for. I also suggested a vitamin supplement, since eye conditions in tortoises can sometimes be related to vitamin A deficiency. The other tortoise was an habitual escapee, continually getting out of her garden into neighbouring properties. She told me a previous vet had drilled a small hole in the edge of the shell so she could tether the animal and keep it safe. Being young, naive and gullible, I agreed to do the same. I made a small hole at the margin of the shell and off the woman went.

Over the next few weeks, I did the same for a few other tortoises and asked her one day if it was working. The answer surprised me and has stuck in my mind. She told me she had threaded thin elastic (knicker elastic, she called it) through the hole and tied it in a knot. After moving away in a straight line from the tether point, the tortoise could go no further and turned to come back. It is an amusing vision but perhaps today it is something I would not condone.

Interestingly, the rules concerning keeping tortoises have changed dramatically since 1984, when European legislation was developed. This provided three species of Mediterranean tortoise (the Spur-thighed, Hermann's and Marginated Tortoise from Greece) with cover under CITES (Convention on International Trade in Endangered Species) regulations, as well as by individual EU or national laws relating to their sale or possession. The Egyptian Tortoise (*Testudo kleinmanni*) was added in 1994. Thus tortoises covered by these regulations may not be sold or offered for sale unless the seller has a certificate issued by the CITES authorities. Anyone who breeds tortoises must also hold the relevant certificates before they can sell any offspring.

In a totally unrelated incident, I had an injured tortoise brought in as an 'out of hours' emergency to Tile Hill (on these occasions it was really useful to live at a surgery). The owner admitted he had run over the animal as he was mowing some long grass with a hover mower. The top of the shell was badly damaged with a portion missing and cracks extending down to the openings for the legs. I decided to try to repair the damage and kept the animal at my home for a few days. With Diane as my assistant, I drilled some fine holes along the cracks and sutured these together with fine wire. After irrigating the damaged area of shell and packing with antibiotic, I then began to fill the area with Isopon, a car body filler. I had already ensured the product I was using did not generate heat when it was mixed. I have to admit that I was pretty proud of the end result, as was the owner and his daughter when they came to collect the tortoise. I saw the tortoise again a week later and everything still looked good, so I arranged one further visit for a month later. Then, when I snipped out the wire sutures, I noticed the fibreglass was beginning to peel away, revealing new shell beneath. Much to my dismay, however, I was criticised by the practice for spending too much time on the case and not charging enough. It was a very early lesson in practice economics and was not to be my last.

During one morning surgery at Binley Road, I called in the final patient of the morning, a white poodle carried in by its owner, a very well-dressed and well-spoken mature woman. She placed her dog on my consulting room table and couldn't look me in the eye. Puzzled, I asked what the problem was. 'She has been licking around her tail all morning and has looked a bit uncomfortable', was her response. Joan took over and held the poodle for me to examine. I lifted the tail, which was wet and blood-tinged, and protruding from her vulva was a puppy's tail, obviously in breech presentation. 'Congratulations', I said. 'She is in the process of giving birth to a puppy'. I assumed the woman would be quite happy but she was just the opposite. Her quiet demeanour was immediately replaced by an angry expression. 'Young man, how dare you', she began. 'My little girl does not do that sort of thing. She cannot be having puppies'.

With that, she scooped up the poodle and marched out of the surgery, into her car and drove off. She never returned and I could only assume the whelping went OK. I was so shocked at her outburst that I never followed up the case and, as we did not have an address, I could not even send a bill for my professional skills. She had effectively accused me of implying that her beloved poodle was promiscuous, highlighting the fact that the bond between an owner and their pet can be a very strong, and sometimes unusual, one.

On another occasion, again at Binley Road, I could see a man sitting all alone in the waiting room, with no sign of any pet with him. Eventually his turn came and he made his way into the consulting room. Before I could say anything, he had bent down and taken off a shoe and sock and, with some difficulty, placed his foot on to my consulting room table. I could see a horrible looking toe with what looked to me like an ingrowing toenail. The man, who I believe was Indian, had obviously seen the word 'surgeon' on the plate outside but perhaps not realised what a veterinary surgeon actually deals with. Luckily, the doctor's surgery was around the corner, so I got him to put his shoe and sock back on and drew him a map to direct him to where he should have gone.

The major daily routine at this practice was in the small animal sector and, being the larger of the two practices in Coventry, it was inevitable there would be a constant procession of routine and elective surgical cases. I observed initially the well-ordered daily routine cat and bitch spays and cat castrations that took up much of the theatre throughput, followed by elective procedures such as orthopaedic repair of limb bone fractures.

Within a very short time, I was given a surgery day once a week but, to my horror, I was to be there on my own, with no other veterinary support as all the other vets were busy elsewhere or were away. The nursing staff were excellent, headed up by Caroline, and gave me all the support they could but I could sense even they were getting a bit exasperated at how slow I was. I had a fairly long list of spays and castrations to deal with but by lunchtime I had made little progress and the list had grown with other cases being referred from the morning surgeries.

After the trials and tribulations of my first bitch spay in Broadway, I was extremely apprehensive about the three I had to undertake. Even in the hands of skilled surgeons, such procedures are deemed to be potentially problematic. The ovaries lie very deeply in the abdomen, often buried in fat in an overweight dog, and to clamp and ligate below the ovary to remove the uterus and ovaries, you have to apply gentle pressure to effectively make a tear in the broad ligament. This ligament contains blood vessels that can potentially tear, and are then out of reach deep in the abdominal content. If they bleed, blood wells up in front of you as it had done with my first bitch spay shortly after qualifying. Just how much gentle pressure needs to be applied comes with experience but I struggled to master the technique. Eventually one of the established vets came back and, realising I was hopelessly behind in the operations list, helped me out.

This routine was repeated for the next couple of weeks and my confidence nosedived. I had mastered cat spays and castrations but that was about it. I decided at that point to opt out of the surgical rota, a decision I never regretted. I did undertake a few more of these procedures in my next job in Devon but the support I received at that small village practice with a slower throughput was much different. I was already making my mind up within six months of qualifying as a vet that small animal work was what I enjoyed the least. Over the remainder of my career I did less and less of it until I focused solely on farm animals for the next 30 years.

One other aspect of the work the new graduate has to come to terms with is out of hours emergency cover, and all new graduates will recognise the stresses this brings in the early days. We had no mobile phones, so there was a need to have a telephone line near the bed with notebook alongside. On quiet nights, there was always the temptation to keep lifting the handset to listen to the dialling code, just to make sure there were no faults on the line. In Coventry, the vast majority of out of hours calls occurred in the time leading up to midnight, and many of these were road traffic accidents.

We were fortunate in that the practice, with considerable foresight at that time, employed an animal ambulance driver, called Andy. He had basic animal first aid training and would be despatched to pick up the animal and bring it back to Tile Hill Lane for me to see. With Andy and Diane helping, we undertook minor procedures, such as stitching wounds, and general first aid procedures, such as immobilising fractures. More serious or life-threatening issues were directed to the main surgery, where I could meet the duty nurse. Whelping bitches were a common problem, with Caesarean operations an awful lot easier than spays.

All out of hours emergency callers were persuaded where possible to bring their patient into my surgery at Tile Hill Lane. It is much easier for a vet to carry out a consultation with everything at hand, than visit the animal's home which often involved crawling under tables to reach, for example, a cat, which might be far more aggressive in its own environment than it would be in a strange place. There is also a limit to how much equipment and medication you can take along.

Most owners fully appreciated our request and Andy was very helpful. If I could sense we were dealing with an elderly owner who could not easily get their pet to us, Andy would collect the animal and bring it to me, sometimes with the owner in the passenger seat. Other owners were, to be blunt, downright obstructive and often quite threatening on the phone. The suggestion they could get a taxi to my surgery was greeted with comments such as: 'Do you think I'm made of money? I can't afford a taxi'. They were quite convinced it would be cheaper for me to visit them at home.

I think, on reflection, there were, and maybe still are, owners who think veterinary cover is similar to the National Health Service, meaning it is free. Far from it, veterinary practices are run as businesses, not charities. There were, and still are, charities such as the People's Dispensary for Sick Animals (PDSA) that will offer veterinary care to those who cannot afford it and we did direct some owners to the Coventry branch if we felt they might benefit. There was also no veterinary insurance during my time in practice, something the profession now strongly advises all owners to take out.

I remember clearly one particularly awkward owner who phoned me around mid-morning on Christmas Day, as I was the duty vet. His dog was coughing and he thought it might have something caught in its throat. I then agreed to see the dog, explaining I lived at the Tile Hill surgery and that I might need to sedate or even anaesthetise the dog if I needed to examine its throat. I then started giving instructions on how to find us (no satnavs then). His manner then changed very abruptly to one of downright aggression. Did I not realise it was Christmas Day? Was I deliberately trying to ruin his day by suggesting he came out in the car just when Christmas lunch was ready? I resisted the temptation to say that he was ruining mine but remained firm and eventually agreed to meet him mid-afternoon. By this time he had calmed down, had obviously realised he had been a bit unfair on me and was genuinely grateful that I had agreed to see him. The dog merely had a throat infection with enlarged tonsils, there was certainly no sign of choke. He left, paid the bill and gave me a box of chocolates as a Christmas gift.

It was on that same Christmas Day that I received a phone call after dark to go to a farm on the outskirts of Coventry to attend a cow having difficulty calving. The calving itself was uneventful but the journey out to the farm was just the opposite. When you are on duty as a veterinary surgeon on Christmas Day, it follows that you do not celebrate by drinking any alcohol and I was totally sober all day and night (my duty ended at midnight). Police patrol cars, however, can be suspicious of anyone driving on Christmas Day, particularly after dark, on the assumption that most of us are at home.

I was driving out of Coventry, well within the speed limit, when a police car overtook me and immediately slowed right down, so I had to brake fairly hard. I signalled, pulled out and slowly overtook, ensuring that I stayed within the speed limit, and then pulled back in again. The police car then repeated its manoeuvre and I repeated mine, by which time I was getting a little frustrated but also unclear about what was going on. After the third manoeuvre, I stayed where I was as the police car drove slower and slower until we were both doing around 15 to 20 mph in a 40 mph limit area. The blue lights then came on, I was pulled over and accused of driving too close to the vehicle in front. I explained that I was a vet and on my way to an urgent call to attend a calving. The atmosphere then changed completely and the police officers were very apologetic, explaining that they were on the lookout for drunks. I was then told to follow them as they escorted me to the outskirts of town, breaking the speed limit on the way. This was the first of two occasions when I received a police escort in Coventry.

One particularly memorable phone call, or series of calls, I received began around 2am, when the phone began ringing by the bed, where Diane and I were both sleeping. The owner very excitedly told me that her bitch was whelping, so I began to take some details thinking that she was in trouble. Just then, I heard someone in the background shout 'another one has just popped out'. I then asked the woman if there was a problem, only to be told that everything was progressing nicely. She had now produced two puppies and the bitch was looking fine. 'Can I ask why you have phoned me at 2am then please?' I asked. The reply was: 'I have this book on dog breeding and it tells me in the chapter on whelping to contact your vet and tell them when whelping begins, so that they can be forewarned of any potential problems'.

I wished her well, put the phone down, turned over and went back to sleep. The phone rang again around 4.30am and, to my surprise, it was the same woman. 'Is there a problem?' I asked, mentally preparing myself to get out of bed for a Caesarean. 'No, just the opposite. She has produced five beautiful puppies and both mum and puppies look wonderful', said the excited owner. 'Can I ask why you have phoned me back', I asked. 'Because that is what my book says', she replied. 'It says to contact your vet to let them know that the whelping has finished, and that they can stand down now'. I resisted the temptation to tell her to throw the book away, or tear out the pages she had been referring to. I wonder how many of my veterinary colleagues in small animal practice have similar experiences of this book?

I clearly recollect one visit I was sent on, as it was quite close to the Binley Road surgery and on my way to my next call. The caller said she was really worried about her cat and didn't want to wait until the evening surgery. I parked the car outside, picked up my bag carrying most of what I might need, marched up the path and rang the front door bell. The door opened only partly (that should have been a clue) and I was invited into a dimly-lit hallway. The door was then shut behind me. I then noticed the woman was still in her dressing gown (another clue) when she ushered me into the living room and shut the door behind her. I was looking for the cat, when I turned around only to be faced with the same woman now stark naked in front of me, with her dressing gown on the floor. Red-faced, I literally ran from the house to my car, drove off and phoned the practice.

Even before I could blurt out my story, the nurse I spoke to said: 'Did she take her clothes off for you? She has done this a few times to visitors to her house, including Andy'. The practice knew this might happen and sent the 'new boy'. It does bring up a serious side, however, and that is the vulnerability of any vet making a house call, possibly a far greater risk today than when I was in practice. With more than 80 per cent of new vets being female there have been a number of campaigns within the profession to keep them safe. They are encouraged not to make lone visits wherever possible, to assess whether the client is known to the practice and, if they do visit, to ensure a third party knows their exact whereabouts, what time they left, and what time they should be returning. Mobile phones make this much easier.

I walked into a potentially nightmare scenario for a young male vet. On this occasion it was quite harmless but a vengeful female could very easily have begun to tear at her clothes and accuse me of molesting her and I would have been in a very vulnerable position. I had no formal training in the whole area of ensuring personal safety but it is of paramount importance. Much of the teaching aimed at our young female graduates has come from the Suzy Lamplugh Trust. This was set up in memory of the young estate agent Suzy Lamplugh, who was reported missing on 28 July 1986 in Fulham, south-west London, after she had arranged to meet a Mr Kipper. She was finally officially declared dead, presumed murdered, in 1994. The trust works with everyone in the community to raise awareness of the importance of personal safety and to provide positive practical guidance that makes people feel safer and more confident. The BVA has taken on much of the advice from this trust in its advice to members.

This was a very mixed practice and I had the opportunity to gain some experience in all its differing disciplines. I had begun to lose interest (or perhaps confidence) in small animal surgery but I was quite happy undertaking endless consultations during surgery time. I was really keen, however, to gain more experience on the farm and equine side of the practice but with a fairly small client base, and one partner who was also keen in this area, I had to grab my opportunities when I could.

As the new vet in the practice, you are often given the easier tasks to carry out and most of my early farm calls were to deal with such cases as a single lame cow, a calf with diarrhoea or a cow needing its afterbirth removing. Not long after I started, however, I was sent on a call to the largest dairy farm in the practice to 'cleanse' a cow. This is achieved by inserting your arm through the cow's vulva and into the uterus to remove afterbirth that had not been expelled at, or shortly after, calving. This is a fairly common problem, particularly in cows that calve prematurely and in those that develop uterine inertia (poor muscle tone, and hence weak contractions) for a number of reasons including milk fever (*hypocalcaemia*), in which blood calcium levels fall and the cow often becomes recumbent as a result. This procedure is normally carried out on day four after calving, by which time the afterbirth can be fairly rotten and you hope your protective glove does not tear as the smell can linger for days!

This was a procedure I had carried out a few times and with which I was quite confident. I recall I turned up at the farm late, as I was still fairly slow, with lunchtime approaching. There is a phrase farm vets quickly become able to recognise and which can be intensely frustrating. That phrase is 'while you are here' and is self-explanatory. You are called to a farm for a particular reason and on many occasions you plan your round to fit in with likely timescales on each visit. These timescales can fall apart, however, if you have a series of 'while you are here' requests to deal with, and this was part of my problem.

I still had other calls to do and a surgery to cover later in the day but the additional task I was asked to carry out while I was there involved around 20 cows that had been held back for me, with yet another new experience to cope with. To sustain milk production it is important a cow produces a calf every year and we refer to this as the 365 day calving cycle. To maintain this cycle, it is important a cow begins to come on heat again, be served and back in calf by around 85 days after calving. Most cows will begin cycling naturally (the term used to describe when a cow has started coming on heat regularly and nothing to do with her performance on two wheels), and are served or inseminated at the correct time. As vets, however, we are often presented with cows showing a variety of infertility problems, such as failure to show signs of heat, failure to conceive even though cycling normally and irregular or persistent heats. It is also important that cows are examined to make sure they are in calf. These were exactly the reasons why these 20 cows had been kept back for me 'while I was there' and were a real mixture of problems.

As I became more experienced, this whole area of work became one of my specialisms but at that time, and having been qualified only a matter of weeks, it was a daunting undertaking. Handling facilities vary from farm to farm but on this one they were good and the cows were all lined up for me, each with their back end facing me. As we walked down the line, cows were either described to me as requiring a PD (pregnancy diagnosis), or as a 'non-buller' (not showing signs of heat), or 'with the whites', (a term used to describe a white discharge from the vulva, suggesting a uterine, post-calving infection). I worked my way slowly (no, very slowly) along the line, pondering each one in turn and what my course of action was to be.

When you have your arm inside a cow's rectum or vagina, literally feeling your way around its pelvic contents, I for one used to look away into the distance with a very discerning look on my face. The period of time I looked away for reduced dramatically over the years but on this occasion my onlookers must have thought I had gone into a trance as I tried to make my mind up as to what was going on, and what I should do and say. Some were straightforward, and I either confirmed pregnancy, irrigated the uterus with antibiotic for my 'whites' cases or injected hormone preparations to cows whose ovaries, based on my palpation of their surface through the rectal wall, suggested either a cyst or a 'persistent *corpus luteum*', a structure in the ovary that can inhibit the development of a normal return to heat.

My problem cows, however, and the ones with the most 'looking into the distance', were the ones that I could not be sure whether they were pregnant or not. It is important that cows are confirmed in calf as soon as possible to ensure that the 365 day cycle is adhered to for maximum production. Most cows were presented to the vet at around six to eight weeks after being served (on most dairy farms by artificial insemination), so you start with an accurate service date. Today, this procedure can be carried out at a much earlier stage using modern imagery techniques such as ultrasound but I had no such luxury. I had to make my mind up purely using my own hand deep in the cow's rectum, feeling the uterus and ovaries through the rectal wall, as I had been taught at college and had the occasional opportunity to try on my EMS placements.

The technique I had been taught, and became very skilled at, was one referred to as 'membrane slip'. If you locate and then gently hold the uterine horn between finger and thumb, you can feel thin membranes (those that enclose the developing embryo and surrounding fluid), literally slip between finger and thumb. If you can feel this, the cow must be pregnant. For various reasons, however, the sensation is not always very clear. This may be because the cow has infection in the womb and is not pregnant. It could also be because the uterine is thickened or difficult to palpate easily due to a rectum full of faeces, or it may be because it is a cow that continually strains. On most occasions, these were simply put down as re-checks, i.e. we would examine again in two weeks, when the pregnancy should be more advanced. I had a number of re-checks but I also had cows that were re-checks two weeks previously and on which I then had to make a decision.

The problem you have is that if you get a PD wrong there are some major implications. For example, if you say the cow is pregnant and she is not, then her calving index will lengthen and she will become non-productive, particularly if no subsequent heats are observed and she is presumed pregnant. Of even more concern is if you state that a pregnant cow is not pregnant. The next course of action is often to inject them with a prostaglandin to literally kick-start her cycles by destroying the *corpus luteal* tissue in her ovary, which just happens to be the body within the ovary that maintains pregnancy. So in effect, if you get it wrong, you finish up causing the cow to abort. I survived the session and apart from the fact I was very slow, I got no further suggestion that I had made any mistakes. I look back at this visit as the start of what became a real passion for dairy cow work and launched me eventually into a career focusing on farm animals, and on cattle in particular.

One very wet and windy day, I knew in advance I had a long, tiring and messy job ahead of me, but when I woke up that morning, I never thought I would be on the verge of being arrested as a suspect mass murderer. One of the farm clients had imported a group of heifers into the UK and they had recently arrived on his farm. None of his cattle had horns as they had mainly been removed during the disbudding procedure when they were calves. However, these imported heifers, around 50 in total, had horns, and as such could not be mixed with the farmer's own herd. Welfare codes make it clear that you should not keep horned animals and animals without horns together, as the horned animals will assume dominance and are likely to injure the more subordinate animals without horns.

My job, therefore, was to remove the horns. It is a procedure we do not take lightly, but in this case, as the heifers had to be integrated into the main herd, it was the only route we could follow. The procedure I adopted was to run the first heifer into the crush, which was designed to hold her still with a yolk that closed down over her neck, leaving her head accessible for me to work on. One of the farm workers then placed bulldogs into her nose. These are metal clamps with two arms, one of which is inserted into each nostril and then closed together over the septum. It has the same effect as the ring in a bull's nose, but the bulldogs do not penetrate through the septum and this is a very effective (and in my view a humane) way of restraining an animal. With the head pulled to one side, I then injected local anaesthetic into the groove behind the eye. This effectively blocks the cornual nerve to desensitise the horn and associated skin and is very similar to the nerve block used by the dentist prior to a filling or extraction.

Once I was satisfied the anaesthetic had worked, I then began the procedure to remove the horn. My preferred approach was to use 'embryotomy wire'. This is multi-strand wire that has a cutting effect if moved to left and right of an object. It was designed for dismembering dead calves during the calving process, another procedure I became very skilled at, and will describe later. By a rapid sawing movement, each horn was removed at its junction with the underlying skin. The main problem then was bleeding, as there are many vessels around the base of the horn that were exposed and spurting blood. Some were in the skin and could be easily clamped off to stop the bleeding, while others were in the horn substance and had to be cauterised with a hot iron.

As I said earlier, it was both a wet and windy day and, although we did have some cover, I gradually became more and more spattered with blood over not only my protective over clothes, but my face, hair (I hate hats) and hands. We had made a very early start and by the time we finished it was past lunchtime. As I was only a mile away from Tile Hill, I quickly cleaned up my equipment and waterproofs, jumped in the car and set off home. As I joined the main road into Coventry there was a sign stating 'traffic census – please stop if requested'. Sure enough, a hand went out directing me into the line of cars being questioned. When I lowered the window, forgetting for a moment what I looked like, the interviewer recoiled quickly and shouted to a policeman supervising the traffic flow to come over. He took one look and ordered me out of the car. Other drivers then looked on in disbelief, for standing in front of them was a man in wellington boots whose shirt, face, arms and hair were covered with matted blood, like a character from the film *The Texas Chainsaw Massacre*. I quickly began to explain who I was and what I had been doing, but I was still asked to open the boot of my car, presumably to check for a body. We all eventually parted on good terms and I went home for a welcome soak in the bath.

I did get the chance to attend to a few horses while in Coventry. These were mainly ponies kept for pleasure and many of the calls were to those with colic. These cases often occurred during weekends and evenings, and as such were treated as emergencies. Most were fairly straightforward 'spasmodic colics' in which increased gut motility results in gas build-up in loops of intestine, which in turns leads to abdominal discomfort. Using injectable spasmolytics to relax the gut wall often provided rapid resolution. Many of these colic cases seemed to follow periods of 'excitement', such as being ridden out over a weekend and thus fed more, after a week stabled.

On the outskirts of Coventry was a small rare breeds farm where many of the more old-fashioned, and hence rarer, breeds of domestic livestock were kept. The farm was open to the public to raise awareness of the species and raise funds to preserve them. The Rare Breeds Survival Trust was, and still is, a national organisation based in nearby Stoneleigh at the National Agricultural Centre. I was sent out to this farm one morning to carry out a number of routine vaccinations, to trim the feet of some sheep and also to rasp the teeth of 'one of the horses'.

The cheek teeth of horses continue to grow throughout their life and, unless there are any dental abnormalities, they grind against each other constantly and wear down the surfaces. If the teeth are out of alignment, however, and the cusps of the teeth are no longer able to grind fully against each other, then the margins begin to become overgrown and can become very sharp. Depending on what part of the tooth is affected, either the soft tissue of the tongue or the cheek can quickly become raw and painful and the horse either stops eating completely or, as in the case of the horse I was asked to see, begins to 'quid', a term used to describe food dropping from the mouth during chewing (and another sure sign of mouth discomfort). Rasping the teeth essentially involves the insertion of a rough file on a handle into the horse's mouth and, by a backwards and forwards movement over the sharp margins, grinding them down. I had carried out the procedure previously and felt fairly confident as I approached my patient, rasp and bucket of water (for cleaning the rasp) in hand. I stopped in my tracks because pretty well the largest and tallest horse I had ever seen was walking towards me, a Shire horse stallion. Bearing in mind I'm a little over 5 ft 8 in high, this was going to be a challenge.

Sensing my slowing step, the owner told me they had made a platform for me to stand on, as they'd had problems previously and there was a need to repeat the procedure every few months. I climbed on to the platform and my patient was lead down towards me. He was incredibly placid and seemed to accept what was about to happen with good grace. There is often a need to use a gag (a metal device placed in the horse's mouth to hold it open) but I was told this was not necessary – or at least had not been necessary on previous occasions. All seemed to be going well, so I picked up my rasp ready for the task. The owner opened the horse's mouth, gently pulling his tongue out to one side, while I slid the rasp down the side of the tongue to the offending teeth, which clearly needed attention. I had hardly started, when the horse's head was lifted up far out of reach and my rasp was left in my hand way below the target. Then began a game which went something like this: tongue out, rasp in, head up, rasp out, with virtually no progress being made. There was no malice, just a simple realisation by my patient that he had the upper hand (or head), and could now very easily control the situation. There was absolutely no point in trying to increase the amount of physical restraint, he was simply too strong for us to attempt anything.

My only approach now was to try to sedate him but with a dose rate that merely made him not care what I was doing to him, but not enough to make him unsteady on his feet and potentially fall over and injure himself. My intravenous dose rate worked perfectly and, with my patient standing with his head bowed in sedative-induced submission, the job was done quickly. I undertook this procedure on the same horse on one further occasion and resorted to the use of a sedative once again. It also gave me a clear reminder of the importance of making notes about cases, in that my diary carried the exact dose rate I had previously used.

My other memorable equine case in Coventry was also the reason for my second police escort as a vet in the city. I was on duty on a bank holiday when I received a call from the police requesting my attendance at an incident near Nuneaton. A pony had fallen into a disused mine shaft that had suddenly opened up in the corner of the field in which it was grazing. The fire brigade was already there but the pony was panicking and it was feared it might have been injured. The officer asked me where I was leaving from and I gave the Tile Hill surgery address. 'We'll be there shortly and will escort you there', I was told and I began to get myself ready, hoping I would not need to destroy the horse as the gun and ammunition were in the main surgery. The police car turned up outside the house and I was told to 'put your foot down, and stay close behind us', which I did, although my ageing Austin 1300 was no match for the patrol car I was supposed to be following. We sped towards Coventry and on to the raised ring road, which had heavy traffic. It was a surreal feeling as the cars parted to let us through. I had my headlights on and stuck close behind my escort.

We eventually arrived at the scene, which had now gathered quite a crowd, including a local BBC news team and camera. The camera pointed towards me as I donned my overalls, over trousers and wellington boots, and marched purposefully towards the hole. I was briefed by the firemen and, as there was not much room in the hole, I was to be lowered down by winch to check the pony. It was then up to me to decide on the best approach. I was given a yellow fireman's helmet to wear and off we went. There was not much room around the pony but that was a good sign as he had not been able to struggle too much. He had a few cuts and bruises mainly on his limbs and underside but I could see no indication of any limb fractures or any other major injury that might make lifting him a problem.

He was still fairly excitable and I decided the best approach would be to give a low dose of sedative to calm him down, but without rendering him totally unable to help himself. The fire brigade had a sling that we managed to pass under the abdomen. I had also fixed a rope head collar with a long lead held by a fireman on the surface and a short lead that I could hold initially and then let go as it was lifted out of reach. Lifting began on my call mainly by hand signals and the pony gradually made his way back to the surface. When the animal eventually re-emerged to a round of applause, he was lowered on to the field and remained motionless and shaking. I was then lifted back out and began to clean up his wounds, stitching those that needed a suture and administering some antibiotic to prevent infection and cortisone to combat stress (a common approach at that time).

I went back home and later in the day sat down to watch the local BBC news, assuming I would have a starring role as the crew had filmed me getting ready near my car, walking towards the hole and being lowered into it. Imagine my disappointment when the only part of me I saw was my hand sticking out of the hole as the pony re-emerged, and the tip of my fireman's helmet. Never mind, it was an exciting experience early in my career, with a successful outcome and very happy owner.

Interestingly, there has been a really good initiative in the past few years to develop a rescue programme for large animals, such as cattle and horses, which become trapped in similar circumstances. This could be in a river, on a cliff face, in a farm slurry pit or in an upturned vehicle on the motorway. The initiative has grown out of work by Hampshire Fire and Rescue Service and has involved much collaborative work with the BCVA and British Equine Veterinary Association (BEVA). Almost every local fire service now has a contingency plan, often with dedicated equipment and trained personnel to deal with these emergencies, and the local veterinary surgeon is usually pivotal to the team.

Another role that I was given responsibility for, as it was close to my surgery, was the day-to-day supervision of the local RSPCA rescue kennels, a role I quickly began to dislike. Every Monday, Wednesday and Friday morning I turned up at the kennels to examine any strays that had been brought in and to treat any minor ailments or injuries that were deemed 'treatable', as the primary aim was to re-home the dogs where possible. As there was limited space, and as strays were a particular problem in Coventry at that time, the kennels filled rapidly to overflowing. At each visit I was told how many dogs I had to destroy that day, each one having been selected because it was deemed to be unsuitable for re-homing due to age, behaviour or 'incurable problems', such as a chronic skin infection, or it had been in the kennels for its allotted time and no one had shown any interest in it. I was effectively the executioner as a steady stream of dogs were brought to me for the lethal injection of barbiturate to be administered intravenously into a foreleg. On some days there were as many as 20 requiring my attention. I suppose on the positive side, they were well looked after and fed during their time at the kennels, as opposed to them scavenging on the streets with the risk of being knocked down or injured by passing cars, but I never really came to terms with the role.

The practice was a busy one and the final aspect of the day-to-day work I was eventually introduced to was the veterinary supervision of greyhound racing at Leicester greyhound stadium, around 24 miles away. The practice had tendered for the work and won the contract some years previously. There were race meetings twice weekly, on Wednesday and Saturday evenings, and a 'trials' meeting on a Monday morning. All of these required veterinary attendance under the rules of racing from the National Greyhound Racing Club (NGRC).

I initially attended two evening race meetings with a more senior vet from the practice. I was very quickly awarded my official NGRC official veterinary surgeon status and began to attend meetings on my own. The Monday morning trials were very straightforward. I did my morning surgery, moved on to the RSPCA kennels and then on to Leicester. I had nothing to do other than attend any dog that was ill or injured during trials, and problems arose rarely. Each evening meeting was considered to be a 'night duty', so in theory I could be home around 10.30pm and then get a night's undisturbed sleep. However, these visits, unlike Mondays, could be very stressful.

The role of the official veterinary surgeon was varied. Some of the tasks were routine and others, particularly for injured dogs, were reactionary. Each meeting began with a pre-race check of all dogs competing that night. They were walked up to me in turn and I was expected to give them a quick once over to make sure they looked bright and alert and were showing no obvious signs of any illness that might affect their racing ability. They were then walked back and forth in front of me to check their gait and to ensure that they were not lame. These inspections were important to ensure that racing was as fair as it could be and that punters did not put money on a dog that might not be race fit. Dogs were also weighed (each had a declared race weight) and identified by ear tattoos. They were all kennelled together in an enclosed area away from the public, although the punters could see them through the wire fencing and generally observe the procedures we were carrying out.

I had very few problems at this stage, with one very notable exception that could have spelled disaster for my veterinary career and local reputation. On this occasion, I had checked all the dogs before the race meeting started and had gone for a quick supper before the meeting itself began (a free meal was my perk). The first three races had taken place uneventfully and I was sitting quietly watching proceedings from inside the kennel when a number of punters started banging on the gate asking to see the vet. This had never happened before and I was still a relative newcomer to these events, so I walked across to see what they wanted. Cries of: 'That number six dog is lame, it should not be on the track', greeted me. Each dog is given a final once over before it leaves the kennel area and goes on to the track. I did notice that this dog had an unusual gait, throwing its hind leg to one side as it trotted but as I knew from its records and discussions with the trainer it had previous surgery on its stifle joint and, as it looked fit and showed no obvious discomfort, I let it go. The swell of dissatisfied punters began to grow and I went out on to the track to have another look with a view to pulling the animal out of the race, but events overtook me and the dogs were placed in the traps ready to go. I was too late and didn't have the confidence to halt proceedings in front of the crowd of several hundred punters. The traps opened and off they went.

I stood on the side of the track with my heart pounding. How was I going to explain that I had messed up to a crowd who had bet their hard-earned cash on a dog I had told them was fit to race? I could hardly believe my eyes when this dog that I feared would come in a distant last actually won the race! The angry group began to move towards me again and I almost turned to run but their whole demeanour had changed. I was being patted on the back and having my hand shook. 'You obviously have an eye for a good dog', was the general feedback and, in a stroke of luck, it spread through the crowd that the new young vet knew his stuff. Little did they know that it was pure luck that things turned out as they did. If I had been more confident, I would have pulled the dog out of the race or made an announcement of its previous surgery and consequent unusual gait. Instead, I panicked and got lucky.

Minor suturing was quite a common request after a dog got injured during a race, often as a result of falling or hitting the side barrier. Another quite common problem involved toe injuries or broken claws, all of which could be dealt with at the track. More serious injuries were rare, although I did have two dogs that collided badly with each other and each suffered a serious limb fracture necessitating euthanasia.

My other role was to investigate potential doping incidents and these followed either a favourite performing badly, or an unfancied dog performing unusually well. Both sedatives and stimulants were fairly easily sourced on the black market, and kennelling prior to races away from trainers/owners and the public, and the veterinary inspections were all parts of the mechanism to keep doping out. We did have a series of doping incidents that I became involved with which were due to the owner doping her own highly fancied dogs and then betting on others. If a doping enquiry was requested, my involvement began with me taking duplicate blood samples for immediate testing for storage, and for the owner if they wished to arrange for their own testing. I then had to obtain a urine sample by catheterisation of males, but by walking around behind a bitch waiting for her to squat. The third sample required was vomit, so firstly I had to get some washing soda crystals down into the dog's stomach, usually administered as I would a tablet, and then wait. Washing soda crystals are a good emetic and within a few minutes the dog will begin to retch. Whatever is brought up is then collected. All samples then had official labels added, which I had to sign along with the owner, who was confirming they were content that those were the samples collected. Then they went off to the laboratory for testing.

One benefit of being the official veterinary surgeon at these race meetings was that I could park inside the stadium in a designated spot. After I realised I could use this spot at other events, Diane and I went along to an evening stock car race and slowly became quite keen on the sport, travelling around to different venues such as Brafield in Northamptonshire, Coventry, Manchester, Nottingham and Bradford. These were the large Formula One stock cars with American V8 engines racing within the BriSCA series, around narrow oval tracks and shunting and hitting one's rivals was allowed. We followed these races between 1974 and 1976, with the stars of the day being Dave Chisolm, Stuart Smith, Dave Hillam and Frankie Wainman. Imagine my surprise, when in 2010 a series was aired on BBC1 called *Tears and Gears* about BriSCA stock car racing and the rivalry, in particular between the Smiths and the Wainmans. I discovered that the two legends of the sport that I had watched 35 years previously were still involved and were now helping their sons towards racing success.

I did have the opportunity to gain experience in a wide range of mixed practice disciplines during my time in Coventry, but I was never really happy in a busy city centre practice. After 18 months, I began to look around for a new job that would enable me to focus more on farm work, a discipline that I was still more interested in.

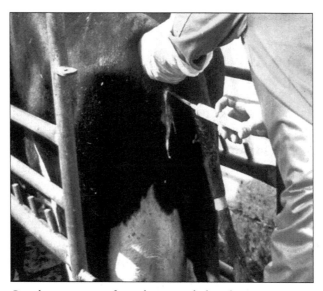

Rectal examination of cows became a daily task!

Chapter 9

It's a Farm Vet for Me – Devon Beckons

Scanning through the situations vacant section of the *Veterinary Record,* I came across an advertisement for an assistant to join two partners in a mainly farm animal practice in the village of Witheridge in Devon, midway between Tiverton and South Molton. I applied for the post, had a very informal interview with the two partners, was offered the job and, as a result, began the veterinary position that was to define my working life for the remainder of my career – namely farm animal work.

I have met and worked with many influential people during my career, but the two partners John Malseed and David Temple, stand out as the role models whom I aspired to emulate. They were very practical, down to earth and hardworking vets who provided a first class service to the local farming community, being highly respected as a result. They nurtured and encouraged me in ways I had never experienced before. Both could be stern and John in particular could be firm, yet retain a 'twinkle in his eye' at the same time, so that I knew when I had made an error, but never felt demotivated as a result. I always learned something new each day.

The job came with a house and car. The house we were given to live in was in the middle of the village, a thatched cottage called Beggar's Roost, across the road from the village hall. The local Mazda garage in the village of Nomansland supplied the practice with its cars and I was given a Mazda 1000. Each car came complete with a radio telephone (no mobile phones in the 1970s). John's call sign was Alpha, David's was Bravo and mine was Charlie. The main base set for controlling our movements was at the practice in Chapel Road, but each house also had a base set and this allowed our wives to keep in touch when we were on weekend or night duty. There were also two phone lines into Beggar's Roost, Witheridge 293, the practice number, and Witheridge 239, our private number, which did lead to confusion at times.

The practice had been established in 1964 and covered a large area of mid Devon, with farms up to the top of Exmoor. When I moved to my next practice after three years, I was replaced by two assistants and the practice continued to grow. It is now named the West Ridge Veterinary Practice and is still essentially a farm animal practice but has companion animal centres in Tiverton, Lapford, Winkleigh and Witheridge and a dedicated equine team. It now has a total of around 14 vets, a significant increase from when John, David and I were working together.

When I worked in the practice most of the clients were small family farms. Some were dairy, some sheep, some beef and many were run as mixed livestock units. The vast majority of the dairy units ran between 30 and 60 cows, although there were two larger dairy farms with more than 200 cows, an unusually high number for that time. Government statistics gathered from successive annual agricultural census figures reveal the average herd size at that time, 1976, in the UK was 39. This has risen progressively to 80 by 1999 and 113 by 2011. In parallel to this increase, there has been a 50 per cent reduction in dairy cow numbers in England and Wales from 2.6 million in 1980 to around 1.3 million in 2011. Much of this change has been the result of smaller farms moving out of dairy production and the remaining farms getting larger, and the number of dairy farms in England and Wales dropped from 28,000 in 1995 to 11,000 in 2010. What was noticeable during my time in Devon was many of our farm clients were at the 'senior' end in age terms, with a high proportion in their 60s and 70s. It has been largely this group who have left the industry and not been replaced.

My first introduction to practice life in Witheridge was fairly typical of how it was to continue, and was a stark contrast from the constant rushing around through city and busy urban traffic desperately trying to keep to time for my surgeries in and around Coventry. The day always began at the surgery with a cup of tea, unless one of us was already out on an early morning emergency. The calls came in and were organised into a daily round for each of us. As I had already gained some experience in Coventry, and particularly as I wanted to impress early on, I made it clear that I wanted to start out on farm calls on my own and not accompany John or David. It is a useful introduction to clients when you accompany one of the established vets in the practice and particularly important for new and apprehensive graduates. However, there is one negative aspect in that you are introduced as the 'new vet' and clients are automatically wary of your abilities when dealing with their livestock. I started off with some fairly routine visits to cleanse cows, disbud and castrate calves and see the occasional sick animal.

When settling into a new practice, a piece of good luck is often welcome and, out of the blue, on one of my first nights on duty, along came mine. The phone rang around midnight and I picked it up and said: 'Malseed and Temple'.

'Who's that?' came the response, to which I replied: 'My name is David Harwood. I am the new vet who has recently joined the practice.'

This was followed by the silence that you begin to recognise as the new boy, before the next inevitable question came: 'Is John or David around?'

'No', I said. 'They are both off duty tonight. How can I help?' They had told me to phone them if I had any problems but I was determined to get stuck into the work of this practice.

'I have a cow trying to calve and it looks as if she's torn herself and is pushing her guts out', was the response.

'Have you been trying to calve her yourself?' I asked, thinking it most likely he had put his hand in and torn her birth canal.

'No', he said. 'I've just got back from a skittles match. I'm the captain of the village team. I just found her like that'.

'OK', I said. 'I'm on my way', after I had got some instructions on finding the farm.

This left Diane in charge of the telephone, something she had never done before as the practice in Coventry had a dedicated answering arrangement whereby calls were filtered and only the urgent ones were relayed to the duty vet. She could call me up on the radio telephone if she was concerned and could phone John or David if other calls came in.

I eventually found the farm. Luckily it was not far from the village and the lights in the outbuildings were clearly visible from the road as I approached. I opened the boot of the car, donned my long waterproof parturition (calving) gown, grabbed my box already stocked with 'things I might need for a calving', and followed the owner to the cow, which was still standing in the corner of an outbuilding.

It is always easier to examine a calving cow while she is standing if possible. It gives you the chance to assess the position of the calf – forwards, backwards or breech – and any deviations of limbs or head from the normal presentation and its relative size in relation to the size of the birth canal. It is more difficult when the cow is recumbent, often in a more inaccessible position and straining against your arm. I could clearly see the 'guts' hanging outside the cow coming through the birth canal but the intestine that I could see was much too small to belong to the cow. It was, in fact, the innards of the calf. This automatically took my mind to my obstetrics lectures and notes. This must be a schistosomus reflexus calf, I thought, as I pushed my hand in to assess what I was dealing with. I traced the intestines back to what was clearly the backbone of the calf and confirmed my suspicion. Schistosomus reflexus is a quite rare congenital abnormality, the exact cause of which is unknown, whereby the spine is essentially bent backwards so the head can be positioned in contact with the pelvis, giving a severe distortion of the spinal column. This abnormality means the chest and abdominal walls do not develop correctly and fail to close over, thus revealing the innards of the calf. This was what was protruding.

As ever with calvings, you often get an audience and with the arrival of a new young vet having to deal with an unusual calving we were quickly joined by other family members. There are two different presentations with this abnormality, what we refer to as 'guts first' or 'feet first'. Luckily, I had the former and easier option to deal with. There was no way this calf could have been pulled through the birth canal intact so the simple answer, as it was clearly dead, was to cut it into two pieces for delivery. I passed a piece of special 'cutting' wire (referred to as embryotomy wire and used in Coventry for dehorning) around behind the bent spine, and then with a sawing action cut through the centre. This grossly deformed (often referred to as a 'monster') calf, then came out easily in two pieces. I checked inside the cow again to make sure there wasn't a second calf and that there was no obvious damage or haemorrhage, which there wasn't, and my task was complete. I cleaned my overalls and calving equipment, washed my hands and arms and set off back to bed feeling pretty pleased with my efforts.

Word travels quickly in a small village and by the following morning both David and John knew about my calving success before I'd had the chance to tell them. Incoming callers who had heard the story beat me to it! For the next few days, I was greeted with the phrase: 'You're that new vet who cut that weird looking calf out of Bill's cow aren't you?' This was the second time Lady Luck had visited me (the first being my lame greyhound incident). If the calving or whatever other problem I'd had to deal with had gone badly, my reputation might have been the opposite but it set me up for a period in my life where my veterinary skills, my confidence and my competence all improved and I really began to love the job.

I wasn't aware of the Devon dialect until I began to encounter words and phrases I didn't fully understand. One example was an utterance which my Devon dialect book described as sounding like the 'shh' at the start of the word 'sugar' but drawing in air instead of exhaling – this signified 'yes, I understand'. I quickly became familiar with this as it signalled an understanding of any advice or instruction I gave on my farm visits. Place names were also pronounced quite differently to how they were spelled. As an example, I visited the villages of Poughill, pronounced Poyill, and Woolfardisworthy, pronounced Wolsery. I quickly picked this up as I had lived in the countryside all my early life and local dialect was something I had grown up with. For Diane, London born and bred, it became a problem. Many telephone messages she had taken when I was on duty were confusing, not only regarding place names but sometimes the animal involved. A 'yore', for example, was a ewe, or the condition from which it was suffering, e.g. 'it's beds out', meaning a prolapsed uterus.

The Witheridge practice was a true rural 'Herriot-like' practice that I rapidly grew into. It covered a large geographical area and overlapped with other practices in the area. South Molton to the west, Tiverton to the east and Crediton to the south marked out our main catchment area, but with some individual outlying farms. I never tired of travelling north, however, as this took me up into the Exmoor National Park. This is an area of true natural and outstanding beauty, where I regularly saw red deer on my travels to and from the practice and outlying farms. Devon's lanes in this area are narrow, often with a bank and high hedge and regular passing places. Locals knew the roads and I had to learn how to drive on them very quickly, sounding my horn on blind spots, and regularly waiting in or reversing back to the nearest passing place. I only had one car accident in this practice and not surprisingly this was a head-on collision in a narrow lane, luckily at relatively low speed. Coming in the other direction (and obviously too fast) was a grockle – the local term for a tourist – and his family. His car was bigger and more robust than my Mazda and came off relatively unscathed but the mudguard and front wing of my car crumpled on to the tyre. After exchanging details, the family continued on their way but I had to get a helping hand from a passing tractor driver, who lent me his sledgehammer so I could redesign the front of my car!

We had no satnav in the 1970s when I began to learn my new patch. Farms were often isolated and difficult to find, many along farm tracks and almost invisible to a passing car. I became quite proficient at using an Ordnance Survey (OS) map, with my notebook full of farm names, addresses, phone numbers and, more importantly, six-digit map reference coordinates. We had a map on the wall in Beggar's Roost, so Diane could keep an eye on where I was during my duty evenings.

The amount of clinical experience I gained in Witheridge cannot be over-emphasised. We met up at the practice at around 8.30am each day, unless one of us was still out on farm from early morning or overnight visits, whereupon John or David allocated the calls to the three of us. John and David both had routine farm visits already fixed, so they dictated the direction each of us set off in. As the new boy, I initially picked up the more widely dispersed visits and after a short time began to get my own farms. At that time, we made far more individual farm visits than vets do today. Farms were smaller and overheads far less, so a visit could be made to cleanse a cow, to examine a lame cow or to a calf with pneumonia. Many such presentations today will either be held over for the next routine vet visit or even treated by farm personnel as farms have increased in both size and staff experience. I would set off regularly from the practice with a list of calls to between ten and 20 farms, giving me an unparalleled exposure to a wide variety of conditions. Modern new graduates may rarely encounter today cases such as wooden tongue (actinobacillosis) or lumpy jaw (actinomycosis). My experience, skill and, more importantly, my confidence continued to grow.

The major part of my time working as a vet in Witheridge was spent out on the farms. The practice did have an evening surgery but this was as different to my previous surgeries in Coventry as one could imagine. My patients were often farm dogs with cuts, broken claws or whelping problems, but could equally include a lamb with a broken leg or a ruptured pig. The routine ops such as bitch spays and cat castrations were booked in and undertaken between farm calls by whoever happened to have finished their round first. After my experiences in Coventry, where my confidence as a small animal surgeon had taken a fair knock, I was relieved that to begin with, I only assisted David or John, eventually taking over the lead after a while so I could take my turn on the operating rota.

Oddly enough, one of my most memorable operations was undertaken in the bar of a local pub. The call was to see a pig with a big lump in its perineal area, which sounded like an inguinal hernia. I had suggested bringing it in to the surgery but the owner was insistent I visited him as the pub was open and he was 'too busy' to bring it in, an excuse I've heard many times over the years. As I had repaired inguinal hernias, or ruptured pigs as they are often referred to, previously I thought it would do no harm to take my instruments with me and deal with it. What I hadn't prepared for was my audience. Sensing that this could be entertaining, the pig, only a small one, had been brought into the bar and was sitting on a towel draped over one of the tables, surrounded by a group of early evening drinkers waiting for the entertainment to begin. Undeterred, I sedated the animal and set about castrating it and repairing the hernia, which luckily went without a hitch. A smile came across my face every time I drove past that pub, and although Diane and I called in a few times for a social drink, I couldn't bring myself to sit at 'that table' whenever we visited.

The practice was at its busiest during the lambing season, when the three of us were at full stretch and often working late into the night or with early morning calls. Compared to the number of lambings modern graduates are called to assist with, I gained more experience in the various procedures needed than they can even dream of. The larger, more intensive, modern sheep units can cope with the majority of lambing difficulties presented to them. Modern shepherds have become skilled in lambing practices and principles and many veterinary practices run regular lambing courses to provide suitable training, so only those requiring a Caesarean are referred. Smaller flocks, and in particular the hobby sheep keepers, will still call their vet, so the modern graduate will still have the chance to lamb a ewe (which is possibly one of the most rewarding experiences for a large animal vet) and the trend in the last few years is to have the ewe brought to the surgery.

In Witheridge, however, the practice policy was to visit the farm, with only a small number being brought into the surgery. On a busy evening, when Diane took over the phones for the night and I was on duty, calls usually began to peak around 7pm, although they had already continued at a steady pace during the day. It was not unusual to have four, five or more lambings being queued (or in modern terminology triaged) depending on perceived urgency.

Diane had been briefed with a list of questions to gauge the urgency of each request for help. I was available on the radio if I was near the car and she could always contact either David or John if she had doubts or felt that I was getting bogged down with calls waiting or urgent calls in the opposite direction to where I was. The most urgent were those where anything was 'showing', particularly if a lamb's head was protruding from the vulva, and these always received priority. Other urgent cases were those where there was excessive blood loss, and those where the ewe was obviously sick, or straining vigorously but producing no sign of a lamb. The less urgent cases were those where lambing had obviously started but nothing was happening. These were mainly ringwomb cases, in which there was minimal cervical opening, or breech cases where no part of the lamb had been presented into the pelvis so the ewe did not strain.

Each presentation had its own approach. With a 'head out', the practice policy was not to 'push it back' if possible as the lamb's reflex efforts may push a limb through the uterine wall, but to slide one's hand down the space between the head/neck and vaginal wall to locate a limb (which was normally facing 'back into the uterus') correcting and then delivering. Ringwomb cases necessitated patience and gentle stretching of the cervix by opening and closing one's fingers inside the cervical opening, which slowly opened up in most cases.

My most sophisticated piece of equipment for lambing comprised a length of washing line passed down through a piece of alkathene water pipe to form a loop at one end. This was invaluable for easing a lamb's head through a narrow pelvis where there simply was no room for my hand to guide it through. It could be placed over the back of the head, behind the ears, and then held firmly in place by the hand outside the ewe, while the other hand located and guided the limbs through the birth canal. If a Caesarean was needed, this was also undertaken on the farm. A makeshift operating table could easily be assembled with four straw bales, which was the right height for me. The wool on the left flank was removed and the procedure carried out under local anaesthetic infiltrated along the site of the incision. I quickly became very slick at the procedure!

Ewes in late pregnancy, particularly if over-fat or carrying multiple lambs, often suffered from a prolapsed vagina/cervix – presenting with a large, fleshy, spherical organ protruding through the vulval lips. There was always the danger this would become damaged and a prolapse also increased the likelihood of infection rising through the cervix, causing the lambs to die. We were regularly called on to replace and retain them. The organ was gently washed clean and with lubricant eased back through the vulval lips. The problem was how to retain it so it wasn't pushed out again.

The solution was simple – the construction of a baler cord harness, which was a speciality of this practice I picked up and used successfully for the remainder of my time in the job. It consisted of three lengths of baler cord, the type used to tie bales in those days and regularly found in heaps on farms, which were used to create a harness over the shoulders of the ewe. It then ran down the back of the animal, around under her inguinal area to be attached to the back strings. A 'string window' was then created around the vulva that would open up if the ewe needed to lamb through the harness – crude but brilliant. As I am presented with veterinary and farming equipment brochures all showing bright shiny innovative ways of retaining these prolapses, I still smile to myself. An equally sound result can be obtained with three lengths of baler twine but I suppose it does look less professional and image is always important in the modern world.

As the majority of the flocks in and around Witheridge began to complete their lambing, the hill flocks up on Exmoor were just beginning. Many of these were the local Exmoor Horn, a particularly small yet hardy breed. Its size meant we undertook proportionately more Caesareans and although the flock was large and the staff very skilled in lambing, we regularly got calls to assist, particularly at busy times.

One such time was the prelude to what I remember as being my busiest day in Witheridge. It began at around 4am, when the Exmoor farm phoned to request assistance. It was flat-out lambing and had around four or five ewes in difficulty that it could not lamb itself. I got dressed and set off. By the time I arrived, I had six ewes waiting, three of which I managed to lamb with my trusty piece of washing line and some additional thin cords. Exmoor ewes are notoriously small, with a narrow pelvis, so some lambings involved applying my 'washing line' behind the head to hold that in place, and slipping loops of cord around the limbs, then eventually guiding the lamb out through the birth canal like a puppeteer with a marionette. There simply was no room for the lamb and my hand. The remaining three were all operated on and by around 8.30am we had caught up. I was offered and ate a good breakfast and then phoned the practice to be told that it was already getting busy and given a list of calls to make in the same area.

These took me up to lunchtime, when I headed back down to the practice, only to be diverted *en route* to a calving at one of the dairy units. The size of the calf legs protruding told me this was no easy job and, after an examination and some gentle traction, it was obvious the only way this calf was coming out was through a Caesarean incision. Luckily I had my kit with me, so I immediately began another Caesarean on a cow, always a more daunting task than the relatively simple procedure on a ewe due to the relative sizes. After completing this operation, I called in again and was then sent on to another lambing, eventually arriving back at the practice around 6pm. Both John and David were out on calls, so I then took evening surgery. Then in came another calving and, although tired and hungry, I set off on this call. I eventually arrived back home around 10pm, 18 hours after I left my bed to respond to the Exmoor lambing call.

Looking back at my time in practice during the 1970s and early 1980s, such long days were relatively common, although perhaps not as gruelling as the example above. There is an analogy between us as junior veterinary surgeons and junior hospital doctors. We were both expected to gain our experience by working excessively long hours and I for one accepted that. The experience and the confidence I gained were immeasurable in retrospect. Today's young veterinary graduates are not expected to regularly work these long hours (nor are their medical equivalents) and there has been a definite move towards ensuring a better quality of life for young graduates, particularly maintaining a good social life. This has been partly driven by the graduates themselves, but also by practices ensuring that, in what is undoubtedly a faster moving world, new employees do not burn themselves out too quickly. This is mindful of the increasing problem of suicide and mental health concerns among the younger members of the profession.

If I were asked to name one task that I missed when I eventually left general practice it would be lambing, the most rewarding time of the year by far.

Farm animal surgery is carried out far less frequently than that in companion animals, mainly due to economic considerations, whereby the value of the animal may be close to the cost of the surgery itself, or conversely its 'salvage value' at slaughter would often be greater. In Witheridge, however, I was encouraged to have a go by both partners, particularly David who had spent some time working in Australia. Often the practice was happy to only charge for results, waiving a charge if a procedure failed or the animal died. This was a popular approach for the clients and an invaluable one for me as my surgical confidence re-emerged after the traumas of Coventry and my skills began to increase.

During the next few years, I became skilled in undertaking Caesarean operations on cattle single-handed. I also carried out a range of differing procedures, including right displaced abomasum repairs through a single left side flank laparotomy incision, rumenotomy procedures to remove wire and other 'hardware' from the reticulum (second stomach), hernia repairs and claw amputations. I even tried my hand at repairing an intestinal torsion in a cow, albeit unsuccessfully, and a caecal torsion also in a cow, successfully.

'Hardware disease', the term used to describe the accidental ingestion of fragments of wire, nails and screws, has remained an interest of mine throughout my career, culminating in a review of the problem in an *In Practice* supplement to the *Veterinary Record* in 2008. These metallic fragments drop into the reticulum, which anatomically lies next to the diaphragm, and around 2 cm from the heart. As the bovine stomach moves and contracts in a cyclical manner, any sharp fragments can potentially penetrate the reticular wall and migrate forward, causing anything from a mild localised peritonitis to life-threatening damage to the heart or surrounding pericardial sac. A modern and successful method of control/prevention today is to encourage the cow to swallow a magnet. This drops into the reticulum and any ingested pieces of metal stick to it, remaining in the rumen.

I was also introduced by David to the art of embryotomy – a procedure used widely in Australia but less commonly in the UK at that time. The technique essentially enables the veterinary surgeon presented with a difficult calving in which the calf is already dead to cut the animal to pieces inside the cow's womb (as I had done in a more simplistic way with my schistosomus reflexus calf) and remove it piece by piece. This avoids the need to undertake a Caesarean operation on an animal potentially compromised by toxins from a dead, decomposing calf. Caesarean operations can also reduce a cow's future breeding potential, in particular if a dead and decomposing calf is present, so the procedure can be invaluable. I used it many times, taking the skills forward with me to my next practice.

One particularly useful indication, was 'hip-lock', whereby you are presented with a cow calving a large calf, half of which is hanging out of the vulva, but the hind end is firmly stuck in the pelvis due to the dissimilarity in size of maternal birth canal and calf. Many of these calves soon die if not identified quickly, corrected and delivered, usually by turning it through 90 degrees and presenting a narrower plane within the pelvis. If the calf is dead, however, the procedure is more straightforward since the calf can be cut in half across its abdomen. A wire loop can then be placed within the uterus between its hind legs, passed back outside and through a purpose-built embryotome consisting of two parallel stainless steel metal tubes fixed close together. These protect the delicate birth canal from the friction created. By a gentle sawing motion, the retained hind end of the calf can be cut into two pieces, which can then be easily removed.

Embryotomy seems to have largely died out among today's graduates, who all seem to opt for a Caesarean if they cannot remove a calf by conventional means. If used correctly, however, it can save a cow from the trauma of surgery and have a positive welfare impact on the management of calving cows, something to which all veterinary surgeons aspire.

The examination of lame cows is a regular part of large animal veterinary work and much of my time in Devon involved struggling to pick up and hold a foot to identify a cause of lameness, or to trim off excess or deformed horn to restore its shape. One new innovation that all three of us learned together was the use of wooden blocks and quick-fixing adhesive – the Technovit system. The idea was brilliant, in that by fixing a wooden block to the sound claw of a lame cow's foot, you raise the painful claw off the ground, such that they can walk 'pain free', weight-bearing on the block. Our early attempts were variable but we all three became more skilled in the procedure. Rather than making it a 'special block fixing visit', as we learned the technique, we eventually carried them in the car with us, and it became part of the procedure used when treating a lame cow on a daily basis. This was, in my view, possibly the biggest innovation in our management of lame cows and in particular the alleviation of the pain that they undoubtedly suffered, with the knock-on effect that they remained productive.

We gained a new farm client while I was in Witheridge by the name of James Robertson, who unbeknown to us at the time was also an author of a series of books entitled *Any Fool Can be a ...*. He admitted from day one that he was a novice dairy farmer and had previously kept pigs. Coincidentally he had written the first in his series of books entitled *Any Fool Can be a Pig Farmer*. I instantly warmed to James and visited his farm many times to examine and treat sick cattle, calve cows, and undertake routine TB tests and blood sampling for brucellosis.

I remember turning up one Saturday morning to find James milking the cows in his herringbone parlour, with one cow down in the pit with him. This should not happen! In the herringbone parlour, the cows stand in two lines either side of a pit, which the milker stands in to give them easy access to the cow's udder. They stand in a staggered fashion, hence the name herringbone. Just how this cow came to be in the parlour was puzzling because there was no easy way out again, and we finished up having to cut through some metal work to release her and then weld the cut ends back together to make a good repair. What was more amusing, however, was that at the end of this exercise, James then said the real reason he had called me out was because of another animal he was concerned about – and not the cow in the parlour! Not surprisingly, this case finished up in his next book *Any Fool Can be a Dairy Farmer* and, although not mentioned by name, I could recognise this incident and others that I had been involved in, including a dramatic description of a prolapsed uterus I had corrected. I knew I was the 'young vet' he referred to.

John, in particular, was very keen on the horse work in the practice and it had many equine clients. We were in the centre of a popular fox and stag hunting area and we did the work for both the Tiverton Foxhounds and Staghounds. As such, I had limited involvement with horses while in Devon but one case I clearly remember occurred during one of my nights on duty. I was out on other visits when Diane received a telephone call from the owner of a pony which had cut its foot and was bleeding. Diane explained that I was out and had been briefed to ask how much bleeding there was and if it were urgent. The owner reassured Diane it wasn't too bad and it could wait for me to finish my other call. I was delayed, however, and Diane phoned the owner back to be told that the pony was still OK, the bleeding had now reduced. When I eventually arrived at the stables however, I was presented with a scene reminiscent of a horror movie. There was blood everywhere and my patient was now so anaemic that I could almost blow him over. It was only a small cut but it had severed a major artery on the lower rear side of the limb. It only took a couple of sutures and a compression bandage to stop the bleeding. We didn't have the resources to transfuse at that time, but the pony did make a full recovery. I know Diane felt awful but, in fairness to her, the owner simply hadn't realised how serious things were getting and my back-up should have been despatched.

My mother and father really enjoyed our time in Witheridge and became regular visitors. The one and only time I took my father out with me was when I was working there. They were visiting one night when I was on duty and I had a call to visit a 'blown calf', one with ruminal tympany, which is literally a gas build-up in its rumen and is both urgent and life-threatening. I knew my father was very squeamish but I asked if he wanted to come out with me to see what I did for a living. He agreed and we set off to a farm I knew well and with owners I really got on with. It was a very emotional experience in retrospect, as my mother told me afterwards that, although he didn't tell me, he was so proud of what I had achieved and how I did my job. It wasn't long afterwards that he became ill with lung cancer and died aged only 54.

In addition to my veterinary experiences in Devon, I also experienced two of the worst extremes of weather I can remember, and so different from each other. The summer of 1976 was incredibly hot and dry, with no rain falling for many weeks. The situation became so critical that domestic water supplies were shut off in the village and standpipes were erected. We had one at the end of the road.

We were told the water needed to be boiled before we could use it as drinking water and you only realise how much water the average household uses when you have to carry it. Everyday procedures such as flushing the toilet, washing dishes and clothes, keeping yourself clean – and I often came home dirty and smelling of cows – use an incredible amount. What was most frustrating, however, was the heavy rain that began to fall a few days after the standpipes were installed. It was not enough to cause our mains supply to be reinstated but enough to get us soaked while queuing to fill our kettles and buckets. How ironic.

In contrast, the winter of 1978 will be remembered in Devon for the heavy snowfall that left much of the county under deep drifts for many weeks and presented major problems for livestock. It also tested our ability as vets to provide the support the animals needed.

It began on a Saturday morning and I was on duty. Snowfall in Devon was not uncommon and each of our cars had either snow tyres or chains kept at the local garage, so my first visit as the snow was beginning to settle was to get my Mazda fitted with chains. I then set off on a list of calls, culminating in one on Exmoor. Conditions began to deteriorate badly by lunchtime, when I finished my last call and headed back south to Witheridge. Suddenly, I was in a complete white-out and I began to realise that I was in trouble when I could no longer see the road ahead or any sign of where I was. I radioed Diane to tell her roughly where I was and agreed to give her regular updates during the remainder of my journey. The chains were brilliant and I kept going through lying snow more than 12 inches deep, with drifts much deeper, hoping that I could avoid the edge of the road and a certain drop into a ditch. After what seemed like an age, I did eventually arrive back home and was the last vehicle to get into or out of the village for the next ten days. I parked my car across the road from our cottage and by morning it was completely buried in snow. All that was visible was the tip of my radio aerial. The snow had reached the top of our back door and halfway up the windows of the conservatory. We were completely cut off as all the roads into and out of the village were impassable. There were drifts 12 to 15 ft deep on the main road through the village and all the approaching lanes with their high banks had filled with snow.

We realised there was no way we could carry on working under such conditions and resigned ourselves to give whatever advice we could to our clients by telephone.

After two to three days, it became clear we were in for a long spell of isolation and we decided we would try to provide whatever help we could on foot. Getting around wasn't easy, but we could walk along the tops of the hedges out of the village and arranged to meet our clients on their tractors, which were the only vehicles able to move around, albeit only on their own farms. The three of us set off in different directions each day, ensuring that we had a companion in case we ran into problems such as disappearing into a drift. Diane was my companion, although for some reason I seemed to be rescuing her rather than the other way round. We did this for the next few days and I was able to calve cows, lamb ewes, and undertake Caesareans where needed – all courtesy of our instruments carried between us in rucksacks. We even featured on the local Devon TV news one evening when we were spotted by a passing news helicopter. Eventually, a huge Komatsu snowplough broke through and at least our main roads were clear but the lanes took a long time to become passable by car.

After three years in the practice, I decided to look around for another position. This was partly due to the rural isolation that I knew Diane felt after being brought up in the centre of London and partly due to the long hours. The practice had continued as three of us but the workload was increasing rapidly. There were days when I would meet either John or David on a farm at 7am to carry out non-urgent surgical procedures, such as repairing a displaced abomasum (quicker with two of us), then continue into a full day of routine and emergency visits and surgeries. At the end of the day, whoever was not on duty would then be returning to the practice at around 7pm to undertake routine small animal operations, such as spays. These long hours undoubtedly put a strain on my marriage and with mixed feelings we decided to move on. I was replaced by two new assistants, and as such, in an ironic way I was quite proud.

My time in Witheridge was hard, yet fulfilling and inspirational, and for that I will always be grateful. It also set me off on a journey that would mean I would specialise in farm animals for the remainder of my career.

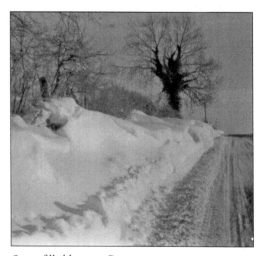

Snow-filled lanes in Devon.

Chapter 10
Over the Border to Dorset

Finding a new post in the 1970s other than relying on word of mouth was solely dependent on looking through the situations vacant pages of the *Veterinary Record*. Today, there are other journals carrying advertisements for situations vacant, such as the *Veterinary Times*, and, of course, both have a strong internet presence. It wasn't too difficult finding a post at that time. In fact, every job interview I went for I was offered, and I don't think this was purely down to my dynamic presence. There were far fewer of us, only 65 in my year at the Royal Veterinary College compared with 250 today. At that time, apart from the occasional overseas vet applying for work in the UK, we did not have the significant influx, particularly from Europe, that we have today.

One advert caught my eye, that for a farm animal assistant to join an eight-vet practice in Blandford Forum, Dorset. Then it was called Cruickshanks, Ellis and Hayward, but it is now known as the Damory Veterinary Clinic. Having made up my mind that I wanted to specialise in farm animal work, the practice immediately appealed to me as it had split its activities into farm, equine and small (companion) animal sectors. All vets specialised in one or the other, although with some overlap during out of hours cover. I also developed an instant rapport with the senior partner, John Cruickshanks, a Scot originating from Kirriemuir. I was offered the post on the spot, and Diane and I instantly liked the area and decided to accept. So in late 1978, after three years in Devon, we moved to Dorset.

We had always lived in practice accommodation in both Coventry and Witheridge but the policy in Blandford was for us to buy our own property and for the practice to recognise this financially. While we looked around for something we could afford as newcomers to the property ladder, we moved into a very small flat at the end of the drive from the practice premises Damory Lodge, known as Ty Bach. This is a Welsh phrase meaning 'little house' and was perhaps an omen for how significant a factor Wales would become in my life from 1983 onwards. We eventually bought our first home, 3 Stanton Close. It was a relatively new house and very close to the practice, so it was easy for me to get to the surgery and even come home for lunch if I had time.

I quickly realised that I had become quite skilled in farm work after my experiences in Devon and I settled into the practice with ease. As ever, it was learning a new area that created the main problem, in particular finding new farms. As in Devon, it was down to finding my farms from six-figure OS map references and marking them on my personal copies for my next visit. This practice covered a wider area than my previous one in Devon with farms spread across around 70 per cent of the county, from the A303 in the north to Corfe Castle in the south, from Dorchester in the west to Salisbury in Wiltshire in the east. This was partly due to the Blandford practice being part of a larger and historical group that eventually decided to separate. When the split had taken place, most farm clients went with their closest practice but others preferred to stay with what was the main practice, namely Blandford. So we finished up with some farms, particularly those around Corfe Castle, that were more than a one-hour drive away, even without the traffic.

Talking of traffic, although it had been an issue at times in Devon, it was a major problem in the summertime in Blandford as some of the main through roads to Bournemouth, Swanage and Weymouth came through our catchment area. Shortcuts had to be followed and some of these even took us across fields and down farm tracks to beat the queues. Urgent calvings on a bank holiday Monday in south Dorset could present major problems.

I did have to take one step back technologically, however, in that the Blandford practice did not possess a radio telephone communication system of the type that had proved so useful in Devon. Instead, we were each issued with a small pot of five pence pieces to use in public payphones. The routine was to set off on your round and phone the practice when you had either completed your calls or when you were heading off to a new area, with a view to picking up any other non-urgent calls that had come in after you had left. If an urgent call came in during the working day, the receptionist would leave messages along your route with farm clients for you to phone in. This worked during the day, when typically four of the eight vets would be out on farm calls. In the evening and at weekends it caused us all many frustrating and irritating problems.

A typical example might be a call to a farm near Wareham for a cow with milk fever, a condition in which, immediately after calving, the cow suffers a dramatic drop in blood calcium and becomes recumbent and unable to stand. This can be life-threatening if not treated. The cow is given intravenous calcium and usually stood up before you left. You stop at the first phone box to phone through to, in my case, Diane to be told that there are no more calls and to head home, a 30- to 40-minute journey depending on traffic. Unknown to you, a call then comes in from a farm that you drive past in blissful ignorance, only to arrive back home and be sent back to retrace your steps. How I missed the radio telephone; mobile phones now make the lives of travelling farm vets much more efficient.

The Blandford catchment area had many large estate farms and dairy units and far fewer family farms than I had been used to dealing with in Devon. As the new boy in the practice, however, I began by spending more time with these smaller farms as the large dairies all had their regular routine visits either weekly or fortnightly, at which all the routine procedures such as fertility and pregnancy diagnosis examinations and foot trimming took place. All the large farms already had a practice farm vet looking after their interests but there was one that had a vacancy and I was given the Fountain Farming dairies. This gave me 500 cows to look after, with a weekly visit to one or both units, and I developed a good working relationship with the farm personnel on both.

Today's dairy specialist vets base much of their fertility work around the ultrasound scanner. This is a probe that is inserted into the rectum of the cow to give a scan of the uterus and its contents, particularly for pregnancy diagnosis. This is a vital part of any dairy management programme, the aim being for each cow to have a calving index of around 365 days, as previously explained. It is important, therefore, for the farm vet to ensure that the uterus is healthy after the calf has been delivered, that the afterbirth has been voided and that there is no residual infection. Ovarian function must then be maintained and any abnormality investigated and treated. Ultrasound scanning was not a widely available tool during my time in practice and throughout my career all these examinations and procedures were undertaken manually using my fingers.

After the hand and arm are inserted into the cow's rectum, it is possible to palpate the reproductive tract through the rectal wall. I had become quite skilled and confident in these procedures, despite my earlier uncertainties in Coventry, and could undertake accurate pregnancy diagnosis (PD) from around eight weeks in mature cows and six weeks in heifers in calf for the first time. This was based partly on the increased size of the uterus but also by a technique I have already outlined called 'membrane slip', in which by applying gentle pressure on the uterine horn between finger and thumb, one could feel the developing foetal membranes 'slip' between them. Ovarian activity could similarly be assessed by feeling the shape and size of each ovary between the finger and thumb, assessing the stage of the cycle and treating accordingly. We now have luteolytic products given in an injection that literally kick-start the cycle by causing the corpus luteum to regress and the cow to display oestrus shortly after. I honed my skills at a time when we manually expressed the corpus luteum between a finger and thumb with the same overall effect but with the risk that a cow could bleed from the ovary if too much pressure had been applied. Luckily this never happened to me.

Looking back at my early experiences in Coventry when my first fertility visits were traumatic due to my lack of confidence and constant re-checks, I now found myself really enjoying this task and getting more and more immersed in the local dairy farms in particular.

Before the advent of computers, most dairy farms kept some form of fertility record for each cow in the herd. Some were better than others but they were mainly on individual cow record cards and with an overall visual herd display on a circular Bray Board or similar on the wall. I realised that I could provide a better and more personalised service to my Fountain Farming client by keeping my own copy of their records in the car with me. They were all written out longhand and enabled me to carry out fertility analysis, something that modern computers can do in seconds. Diane helped out by copying rough notes into my folders. I began to get involved with management meetings on these farms, discussing with the manager, dairymen, nutritional advisors and others the way forward. I was becoming, and felt, a valued member of the farm team.

Long PD sessions were quite common and to prevent my right arm from seizing up due to the constant pressure of the anal ring and rectum, I began to develop an ambidextrous approach. On one particular estate, I was asked to PD 200 heifers in an afternoon. All had been running with the bull and were at different stages of pregnancy. I was asked firstly to confirm they were in calf and then, by assessing uterine size and presence of a foetus and its size, to give an approximate calving date so that they could be grouped together for management purposes and specific feeding regimes. As I was invited back in successive years to this same farm, I must have been fairly accurate. Incidentally, it is a great way to keep your arms warm on cold days.

I also began to realise that my 'have a go' attitude towards calvings using embryotomy and Caesarean operations where necessary were going down well both within the practice and with the farm clients. The practice policy, at least from the top, had been to send cows that could not be calved conventionally off as 'casualty slaughter' cows. That seemed wrong to me, so I continued with my approach and with a fair amount of success. Although initially I only worked at Fountain Farming, I was visiting all the other large estate farms for other non-routine procedures, such as calvings, cases of prolapsed uterus and other farm emergencies, and I began to become known among the clients. As assistants moved on or new requests for routine visits began to develop, they fell into my lap, and after three to four years I was undertaking the bulk of the routine work on six of the largest dairy units in the practice.

One of my routine visits was to the Crichel herd of pedigree Holstein Friesians, which had built up over many years and was well known in the cattle show world. Such was the value of some of these cows that we were called in to attend even minor problems when they were calving. I was met on a number of occasions with a comment along the lines of: 'Don't forget, if this is a heifer calf, she'll be worth x thousand pounds'. I'm happy to report that it made no difference to my overall approach, although I did perhaps heave a louder sigh when the calf was eventually born alive than I would normally.

A technique now popular that was in its infancy during my time in practice was embryo transfer and it began to be used on this farm. This technique allows us to superovulate a cow of high genetic merit by hormone therapy, so that instead of the single egg she would normally produce, her ovaries produce many more eggs. These are harvested and fertilised in the laboratory prior to being implanted into the uterus of other cows or heifers to grow to term. By these means, many high genetic merit calves can be born to a single high genetic merit cow. Although the donor cow is itself of high genetic merit, the recipient females can be of any genetic status, although they have to be well grown and pass very rigorous health screening for infectious disease.

I became quite heavily involved in the process at all stages, including clinically examining and blood sampling recipients to confirm they were fit, healthy and as free of infectious disease as they could be. I also took part in the administration of the hormone programme to the donor cows to initiate the hormone surge needed to stimulate overactive ovarian function. During one later programme, a number of calvings had required our intervention. Some calves survived but others did not and from memory only around half of the successful pregnancies resulted in a viable calf. As the following programme had resulted in around eight successful pregnancies in donor animals, and to offset the possible loss of calves due to dystocia or difficult calving, we were asked to undertake elective Caesarean operations around 10 to 14 days before the due date. As a result, I undertook eight Caesarean operations over two days with assistance from other practice vets and we had a 100 per cent survival rate of both cow and calf.

One particular bull on this farm known as Crichel Starlight had won many coveted awards in the Holstein show world and was huge, with my eye line level with his shoulders. He was a fairly docile bull but his sheer size did make it difficult to undertake even routine procedures, such as foot trimming. Our best approach was to heavily sedate and 'cast' him, so that he lay down and gave me reasonable access to his feet. We used a sedative known as Rompun (active product xylazine), which was largely given intramuscularly to achieve a degree of sedation in fractious animals. It could also be given intravenously but with a warning that it could cause a rapid lowering of blood pressure and the animal could collapse. I had used the product intravenously on many occasions, giving a small dose into the coccygeal vein that lies on the under surface of the tail, with access gained by holding the tail vertically.

One such occasion is clearly etched on my mind. We walked Starlight into the crush (a cattle handling device), I lifted his tail and injected the usual amount into his tail vein, as I had done several times before, and the gate was opened to walk him out into the yard. He took one or two steps before collapsing half in and half out of the crush. There was immediate panic among the farm staff – this was their prized champion bull and this so-and-so vet had killed him. I was also beginning to panic inside but I had done this before with no previous problems. I then heard a clear and calm voice coming from somewhere saying: 'Don't worry, he'll be fine, he's just fainted after the injection. He'll be round in a moment, it happens occasionally'. The voice was my own, but at that moment I felt as if I was a bystander panicking with everyone else. He did come round quickly, with the added benefit that he was already sitting down, so we quickly trimmed his hoofs while he was still dazed.

This wasn't the only time that Starlight raised my heart rate. During the warm summer months one year, I had a message relayed to me to get to the Crichel herd as soon as I could as I was the nearest at the time. When I arrived in the bottom yard where Starlight was usually housed, I realised he was in trouble by the gaggle of farm staff and the owner waving me over. Starlight was obviously in great distress. He was foaming at the mouth and rolling his eyes in panic as his breathing was becoming increasingly more laboured. What on earth had happened to him? The initial feeling when I arrived was that he was choking on something. Dealing with choke in such a huge, visibly distressed animal without compromising him further seemed problematic, to put it mildly. I decided to try to coax him into the crush to examine him more easily, and I knew this crush dismantled easily if he did collapse while he was contained within it. While walking behind him, I noticed a rapidly increasing rash spreading across the thin skin around his scrotum. This had to be an anaphylactic shock reaction and his behaviour all began to fit. Luckily, I had some adrenaline in the car and gave him the maximum dose I could intravenously into his tail vein. I then stood back with everything crossed. Within minutes he was visibly improving, his breathing became easier and both he and I began to relax. I checked on him later in the day and he was back to normal. I never discovered the cause but the general feeling was he had been stung by a wasp or bee, possibly taking one into his mouth while feeding.

My skills at calving cows, undertaking Caesarean operations, replacing prolapses and repairing a displaced abomasum began to be known around the practice clients and I was actually receiving specific requests to attend. Even though I was only still an assistant and not a partner, I was also being asked to go out to assist new young graduates and troubleshoot when problems arose on clients' farms. I loved this practice, and in particular loved the opportunity to specialise in farm work, with only the occasional small animal surgery on my duty nights and weekends to deal with. I admit to getting out of this whenever I could and relished any farm call that came in during my duty periods, which gave me an excuse to leave the consulting room.

One of the largest dairy units in the area was at Chilbridge, near Wimborne, with nearly 500 cows on a single site. This was very large at that time but small in comparison to modern dairy production, in particular the so-called super dairies. The farm was well known within the practice for being fairly self-sufficient and only calling us in when there was a real problem. It was also what is referred to today as an open farm, one that allowed the general public to visit and observe its activities. Due to its proximity to Bournemouth and the tourist areas along the south coast, the farm received thousands of visitors a year at that time. It had viewing platforms over calving boxes and a large rotary carousel milking parlour, a 'merry-go-round' parlour in which cows stood facing outwards with their udder facing inwards and the milking procedure was carried out from the centre. Visitors could bottle feed calves, generally walk around the farm and were taken out into the fields by tractor and trailer. I had undertaken a number of fairly tough calvings at Chilbridge and had also been watched examining lame cows, disbudding and castrating calves and examining sick animals by visitors as the word quickly got around that there was a vet on the farm. The farm staff were very good at keeping the public away from potentially controversial or distressing procedures, and although a cow calving naturally was a popular sight for visitors, pulling calves out using calving aids or pulleys might have been more distressing.

I remember attending a calving on one of the better cows in the herd on an August bank holiday, when the farm was heaving with visitors to the point that I had to queue down the drive to get in. I eventually got to my patient and realised I was not going to deliver this large calf easily. After some gentle traction, I decided that a Caesarean was the only option and although the farm rarely opted for this approach, on this occasion due to the value of the cow they agreed. I was then asked if I minded the public watching. This sounded a bit daunting but I agreed so the cow was moved to a calving box where there was a long viewing platform. I set about my usual routine for such an operation, cleaning the flank, then shaving up and administering the local anaesthetic. Luckily, the operation went very smoothly and, to a round of applause and loud cheering, the calf eventually made its appearance through the left flank of the cow. I cleaned up, came out the 'stage door' and went out to my car, which was surrounded by farm visitors who had just watched the procedure. I finished up signing a few autographs – a totally surreal experience.

My 'have a go' attitude also surfaced when faced with another problem at Chilbridge, when a cow's head became trapped and partially crushed in the rotary parlour mechanism when the safety stop had failed to work. The cow's eye had ruptured and much of the bone surrounding the orbit was also fractured. Although I knew the procedure for eye enucleation (removal) in small animals, I had never heard of it being undertaken in cattle. The farm was keen to try something, so I agreed to have a go. The cow was deeply sedated and I administered local anaesthetic into the orbit behind the eye. I also undertook nerve blocks to the surrounding tissue, including the eyelids. I approached the eye removal after consulting my college notes and small animal textbooks. I followed a standard approach by suturing the eyelids together over the eye, then gradually dissecting through the various muscle attachments and clamping off the arterial supply. After removing the eye, I then continued to remove any fragments of loose bone that were evident. The socket was then packed with antibiotic powder and filled with a folded bandage, with the end protruding from the edge of the incision. A length of this was cut off each day as the space that the eye previously occupied was slowly filled with scar tissue. The cow made a fantastic recovery and was back at full milk production within 48 hours.

Following this success, I removed several other eyes from cows. These mainly had severe and intensely painful ulcers, most of which had ruptured the eyeball – a potential sequel to the infectious condition referred to as New Forest eye or, more correctly, infectious bovine keratoconjunctivitis or IBK. This bacterial condition is spread between cattle by flies and can be a serious welfare problem on affected farms. Dorset experienced a particularly bad season one year, with many farms and countless cases occurring. There had been a new approach to treating the condition that we all began using. Previously, we had squeezed antibiotic creams into affected eyes or 'puffed' antibiotic powder over the surface, with variable results. The new approach was to inject a small volume of antibiotic under the conjunctiva on the upper eyelid. The antibiotic would then literally 'drain out' through the needle hole and continue to bathe the surface of the affected eye for a much longer period than ointments and powders would remain active. Enucleation was a last resort but from a welfare perspective the intense pain of a deeply ulcerated or ruptured eye could be removed with the eye. This could be easily demonstrated by monitoring milk yields as these returned close to previous levels within one to two days post-surgery, and cows with only one eye can survive very well.

As I mentioned earlier, the roads around Blandford were busy particularly during the summer holiday periods. I received two phone calls from the police to attend road accidents in which animals had been injured during my time in Dorset. One of these involved a horse that had escaped on to the busy Blandford to Salisbury road and was lying motionless on the carriageway having been hit by two cars. I had been told to meet a patrol car waiting for me and to follow it with its blue lights flashing until we reached the scene. As ever, there were many observers around. It was obvious the horse was severely injured and needed to be destroyed. In anticipation, I had brought along the practice gun, a free bullet version. Realising this could result in ricochet from the road surface, the public were moved away from the area until I had done the deed. The horse was then removed and the road reopened.

Another early hours call was far more harrowing. A group of heifers had escaped from their field during a wet and windy night and had taken shelter in a cutting, which just happened to have a railway line running through it. A train driver had reported hitting something and found blood and other body tissue over the front of his train when he stopped at the next station. All emergency services had been called as it was not clear if this were a human or animal tragedy. I arrived after the fire engine but before the ambulance to a scene of utter carnage. There were dead and mutilated heifers, badly injured heifers and unscathed heifers at the scene. I destroyed the worst affected and, having a fair suspicion of where they had escaped from, I gave the possible owner's details to the police and left. However, the scene in that cutting did haunt me for some time afterwards.

Although we tried, we could not solve every problem faced. It was while in Blandford I began to develop a really good working relationship with the government organisation that I would subsequently work for in the remaining 30 years of my professional career. This was the Veterinary Investigation Service, as it was known at that time, and my local laboratory was in Langford in the Mendips. It was to this facility that many of our specimens and samples were sent for testing and post-mortem examination. The veterinary investigation officers (VIOs) were always available for case discussion and I found their help invaluable. I formed a good working relationship with Norman Todd, the senior vet at Langford at that time, who would eventually provide me with a reference when I applied to join the service.

I had one particularly severe and intractable pneumonia problem on a large bull beef unit just outside Blandford. Having tried a variety of measures to improve ventilation and general calf management, we arranged for Norman to come down to the farm to assess the situation. He arrived with a colleague from the university (on the same site at Langford) with an interest in building design and ventilation called Christopher Wathes, who later became professor of animal welfare at the Royal Veterinary College and chairman of the Farm Animal Welfare Council (FAWC). The partnership worked well and the problem did improve slowly after their advice had been followed. The other inspirational partnership that steered me to change career direction was Phillip Francis and John Stanley, a VIO and dairy hygiene consultant respectively, who undertook joint visits to investigate mastitis breakdowns on problem farms.

It was also in Blandford that I joined the British Cattle Veterinary Association (BCVA) in 1978, when it was still a young society. It was a specialist division of the British Veterinary Association and its membership was made up of like-minded veterinary surgeons with a specific interest in the health and welfare of cattle in the UK. I was eventually elected on to its council in Edinburgh in 1996 and served as president in 2002/3.

I had joined the Blandford Round Table during my time in the town and began to make many close friends and became part of the community as a result. This was a real bonus for Diane, who had also joined Ladies' Circle, as for the first time we were able to develop a close-knit group of friends with similar interests and aspirations. Our social life increased dramatically, since in addition to the formal Round Table and Ladies' Circle meetings, we became involved in a constant round of parties, dinners and barbecues. I was often on duty, so call-outs were inevitable but accepted as part of my job. My host knew his or her phone number would be the emergency contact for the vet practice when I was there. I used to take a change of clothing with me, my car containing the equipment was parked outside, and an evening on orange juice was to follow.

A dramatic change of circumstances could suddenly develop during such an occasion. As an example, we were at a Christmas party at a friend's house. It was cold and snowing outside, but the festive spirit, hospitality and warmth were palpable in the house. Then, around 9pm, the phone rang and when I answered a farmer said, 'Sorry to bother you, David, but I've just found one of our suckler cows in a ditch and she's trying to calve. Can you come and help please?' So, after changing into my work clothes, I left the warmth of the house and went out into the snow for my drive to the farm.

Sure enough, my patient was lying in a ditch full of water. The calf's head was out but was only just above the surface. If we tried to haul her out, the calf would probably die or drown – and with a suckler cow, this calf is the main economic product. If it dies, then the cow has been kept for a year with no return. I took my coat and jumper off and, leaving my arms bare, donned my parturition gown and waded into the water, quickly feeling very cold. Luckily, the calf came out fairly easily and was pulled back up the bank to safety, followed by the cow after we hauled her out with a tractor and length of rope. By the time I got back to the party, it was still in full swing but I was cold and rather smelly and was urged to take a shower by the host. I then returned to the party stone cold sober at around midnight, when another calving came in. At that point I just gave up and left my wife to enjoy herself.

On more than one occasion, I was also called out of Round Table meetings at The Crown Hotel in Blandford. These normally followed the same format: a meet in the bar, a three-course dinner and an after dinner speaker. The hotel staff knew my predicament well and if I had to leave on a call, or had told other Tablers I would be late, they would keep my meal warm for me. On two or three occasions, I sat eating my three courses after everyone had finished. I served as social secretary for a year and remember booking a then unknown entertainer. This was Jethro the Cornish comedian, whom I sat next to during the meal. He was, and still is, brilliant. The last time I saw him was at the Mayflower Theatre in Southampton, where he performed to a packed house.

The Round Table introduced me to a group of like-minded individuals who knew how to have fun but who were also heavily involved with a variety of charitable initiatives in the community and in a wider context. One such local initiative was holding a Christmas event for disadvantaged children in the area. One year we asked Harry Corbett of Sooty and Sweep fame if he would be our star guest as he lived nearby. He had retired from his long-running TV series in 1976 and was replaced by his son Matthew, but he was still very active and came along with Sooty, Sweep and Soo, together with his wife. They were so professional in the way they brought these famous puppets to life and the children loved it. The other attraction, mainly for audience participation, was *The Birdie Song* with its accompanying dance actions, which were to be led by three Tablers including myself. So, dressed in red tights, a yellow costume and bedecked in feathers, I jumped on stage with Harry Corbett and his puppets while we all did the routine.

During my time in the Round Table, I also played Agnetha from Abba in our male-only version of a tribute band and, wearing very little, I also did a balloon dance routine at a Round Table ladies night.

Our first daughter, Madeleine, was born on 22 September 1981, exactly one month premature. Diane and I had been away at the BVA congress in Exeter and arrived back in the early evening, whereupon I took over the phones for the night duty. Diane went into labour at around 5am, so my first task was to drive to the surgery, leaving my wife on her own while I phoned my back-up colleague and transferred the phones to him. Then I set off for Dorchester Hospital, where Maddy was born.

John Cruickshanks had retired in 1983 and I was confident that, being the senior assistant at the time, I would be offered a partnership. However, I was dealt a blow when it was offered to a more junior assistant who had a penchant for the small animal side of the practice, which the two remaining partners wished to enhance and establish. It was made clear to me my position was then difficult, as an assistant who I had previously helped and bailed out of problem farm animal cases was to be my new boss. I was also told there were to be no future partnership prospects.

I contemplated setting up my plate, urged on by a number of my very loyal and supportive large dairy clients, but I came up against some legal restraining orders from the practice prohibiting me from practising within a specified area that included half of Dorset. With a newborn baby, I was reluctant to run up large bills by launching headlong into a legal battle with the practice, so I decided to look for another avenue of employment while the dust settled, with a long-term view of returning in 18 to 24 months and setting up my plate.

For a variety of reasons, this never happened and a chapter in my life closed for ever. I decided to move away from the general farm animal practice that I loved so much and into a new area of work.

While we lived in Blandford, I also lost my father; he was aged just 54 and died after a two-year battle with lung cancer. He survived for just one year and two days of Maddy's life.

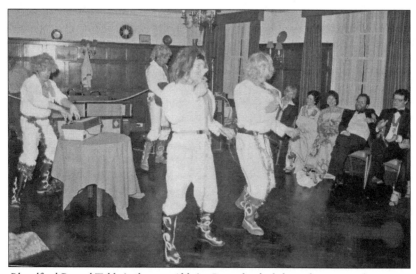

Blandford Round Table 'tribute to Abba' – I am the dark-haired singer in the foreground!

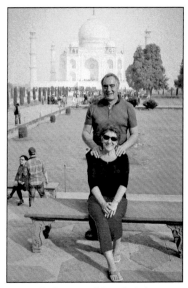

My wife Gerry and I on holiday in India in 2014. (Ch. 17)

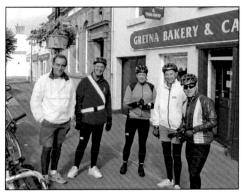

My fellow cyclists on the 'Tour de Vets' charity cycle ride. (Ch. 17)

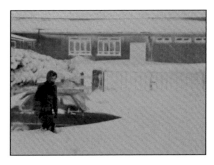

My car amost buried in the snow in Devon. (Ch. 9)

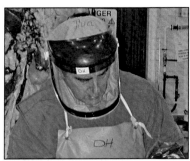

At work on a TB post-mortem examination wearing personal protective equipment. (Ch. 11)

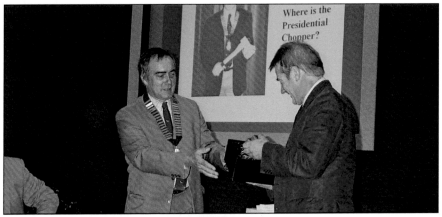

Taking over from my predecessor Dick Sibley (right) as President of the British Cattle Veterinary Association (BCVA) in 2002. (Ch. 15)

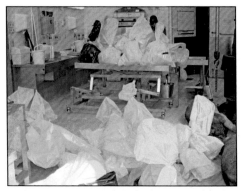

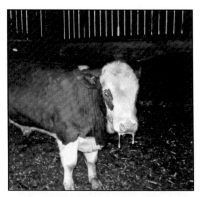

The Monday after the confirmation of highly pathogenic avian influenza in a swan in Scotland – each bag contains wild birds for post-mortem examination in Winchester. (Ch. 15)

A typical FMD case – note the salivation around the muzzle. (Ch. 14)

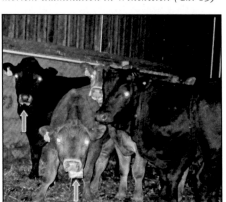

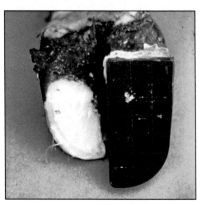

The Technovit system for applying blocks to the sound digit to protect a painful claw. (Ch. 9)

Typical FMD signs in a group of cattle – note the salivation highlighted. (Ch. 14)

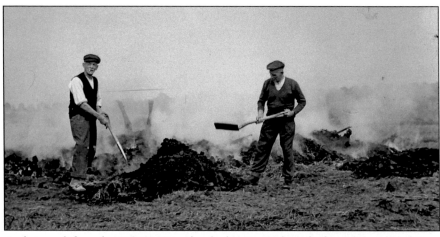

A photograph from the 1967 FMD outbreak, showing work on the funeral pyre. (Ch. 14)

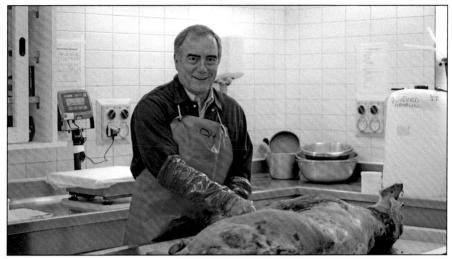

Me at work in the post mortem room at Winchester AHVLA. (Ch. 11)

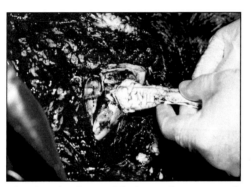

The obex (hind part of the brain) being removed through the foramen magnum at the base of the skull of a cow. (Ch. 13)

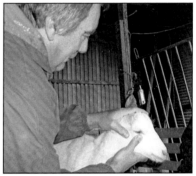

Out on farm investigating a goat health problem in SE England. (Ch. 11)

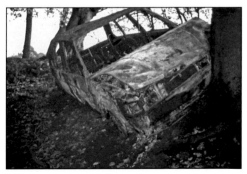

A burnt out ('torched')car; the molten battery material contained high levels of lead, and killed cattle. (Ch. 12)

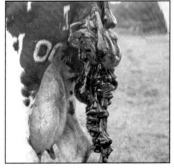

A schistosoma reflexus calf with its intestines hanging from the birth canal of the cow – similar to my first calving in Devon. (Ch. 9)

At work on a TB post-mortem examination wearing personal protective equipment. (Ch. 11)

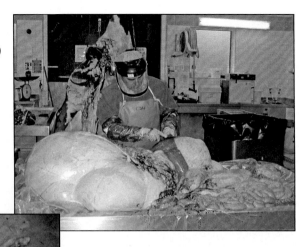

Cow ready for post-mortem examination at Winchester. (Ch. 11)

A schistosoma calf I examined at post-mortem many years later. (Ch. 9)

An adult male lion that had died from chronic interstitial nephritis. (Ch. 12)

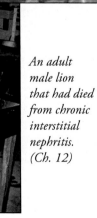

Chapter 11

A 'Man from the Ministry', and Back to My Studies!

After being in practice for almost ten years and confident I was now a skilled and competent large animal vet, I was still only an assistant and having to contemplate starting all over again in another practice. It was perhaps time to reconsider my future.

Having experienced work in the Veterinary Investigation Service as a student at the Worcester laboratory for two weeks during my training and having had dealings with both the Starcross laboratory at Exeter when in Witheridge and more recently the Langford laboratory in Bristol during my time in Blandford, I was familiar with the basics of the organisation. It did appeal to me and I arranged to go up to Langford and sit down with Norman Todd to get a better insight into the job of a veterinary investigation officer.

At around the same time, an advertisement appeared in the *Veterinary Record* for recruitment into the State Veterinary Service (SVS) as either a veterinary officer (VO) undertaking farm legislative activities on behalf of MAFF (the forerunner to Defra) or as a VIO. I had no real interest in the former, so I filled in the application form crossing out any reference to VO. It did not state where the vacancies were, only that they were at a number of locations throughout England and Wales. My application was successful and I was called for interview in London before a board of four senior MAFF vets. I received a fair grilling as a result, from everything related to my practice experience to my thoughts on disease control policy at that time.

The interview must have gone well as I was offered the only VIO post available at that time, in Carmarthen, west Wales. This presented Diane and I with a real dilemma. We both felt that to progress we had to leave Blandford, yet both of us had some of our happiest years together in this Dorset town. We decided to accept the offer but reassured ourselves that it would be a temporary move. I could get some additional experience in a different discipline, the dust could settle and we would return to Blandford after 18 to 24 months. This never happened, however, mainly due to the major increase in house prices in southern England compared with the much lower and relatively stationary house prices in west Wales. The difference between the two was insurmountable and we could not return and remain financially viable, so we decided to stay and I got stuck into my new career.

So it was that on 1 March 1983, I set off early from Blandford for the long drive and my first day in Carmarthen and a new veterinary career. I arrived at around 8.30am and as I headed for the laboratory, I couldn't help noticing that the majority of the children heading for school were in Welsh national costume and I began to wonder what on earth I had let myself in for. This was certainly not what I had expected. What I hadn't realised was that 1 March is St David's Day, the one and only day in the year when the costume is worn to school. On the following day they were all back in their ordinary school uniforms.

Having become familiar with the Devon dialect, I then had to come to terms with living in a part of Wales where Welsh was the first language for many, in particular within the farming community in which I would be working. I was never a linguist and quickly realised what a difficult language it was to learn and pronounce. I cannot emphasise enough, however, just how welcome I was made to feel, particularly by my new colleagues in the veterinary investigation centre in Johnstown, Carmarthen.

Almost without exception, they were all primary Welsh speakers and I knew that Welsh was the language used throughout the laboratory. That was except whenever I was involved in a conversation, or even walked into a room, when they switched effortlessly to English. That ensured I never felt left out or isolated. I could pick up odd words in conversations, particularly when TV programmes were under discussion, for example *Coronation Street* would be said because not every word or phrase has a Welsh equivalent. There were two Toms working in the laboratory. One was referred to as Tom bach or little Tom, and the other Tom mawr or big Tom. They both helped me with pronunciation and spelling, particularly of farm names and villages. I realised I would never be able to learn the language itself but made a conscious effort to pronounce whatever I could. This was invaluable when I asked for directions or wrote down names and addresses while taking histories from the farmers who consulted me.

I only had two occasions in the 11 years I worked in Carmarthen when my inability to speak Welsh was a real problem. One was when I visited a farm in mid Wales to investigate an outbreak of salmonella infection in a herd of suckler cows. Part of the visit was spent taking a history of the farm and the disease incident as the investigation was semi-official, with information gathered and used in the annual salmonella summary produced by government. The data was also shared with the local medical authorities as salmonellosis is a risk to human health. The isolated farm was owned by a fairly elderly gentleman and his wife, both of whom were primary Welsh speakers. This wasn't usually a problem as conversations were invariably conducted in English for my benefit. However, this couple had very limited English vocabulary. They were not being awkward, they simply lived their lives through the Welsh medium and I found out later they did not own a TV set, listening only to Welsh language radio. This was a problem but luckily they had a teenage granddaughter who by chance called in to see them on her way home from school and acted as my translator and intermediary.

The second occasion was more frustrating and could have got me into trouble, but luckily didn't. It was a Friday afternoon and I was the only vet working in the laboratory that day. A dead lamb was brought in for post-mortem examination by a local farmer, whom I later found out, was a prominent member of Plaid Cymru, the Welsh nationalist party. I met him in reception to take a history, apologising by saying 'dim siarad Cymraeg', a phrase I had learned that means 'I don't speak Welsh'. I expected him to revert to English, which was the normal approach when I was involved. He didn't, however, but kept speaking Welsh to me despite my protestation that I didn't understand him. I also kept telling him I was more than willing to do whatever I could to help him find out why his lamb had died but I needed some basic information. In frustration I told him that, as we were getting nowhere with our conversation, he should take his lamb away. I fully expected him to accept that he had made his point and then we could carry on. However, he did just what I suggested – marched out the door, jumped into his Land Rover and drove off, taking his lamb with him. I anticipated I would get a stern reprimand from my seniors, feeling sure that he would make a formal complaint against me through his political and farming affiliations, but nothing ever came of it. Tom mawr did tell me afterwards that he knew the person concerned and that he could speak English as well as I could, but was simply making a point.

I began my Carmarthen job by staying in local hotels, leaving Diane behind with Maddy in Blandford to complete the house sale. Our furniture went into storage but Diane and Maddy joined me soon after in a rented house in Llandeilo. We later bought our first house in Wales in Bronwydd, called Neuaddlwyd cottage, which was on a hillside overlooking the Gwili steam railway and close to Carmarthen.

The origins of the State Veterinary Service (SVS) can be traced back to the 1860s when a veterinary department was set up as a temporary measure to deal with an outbreak of the cattle plague rinderpest. This led to the formation of a government veterinary service, which has continued in one form or another ever since. The Veterinary Investigation Service (which later became the Veterinary Laboratories Agency or VLA) can in turn trace its origins back to 1894, when its forerunner the Central Veterinary Laboratory (CVL) was established in a small basement room in Whitehall, London, to deal with a swine fever epidemic. This remit was widened quickly and, after several changes of location, the laboratory moved into its current headquarters at Weybridge in 1917, one of the first purpose-built veterinary laboratories in the world. The site is still known as Weybridge today and houses an ultra-modern and purpose-built laboratory.

I continued to work in this organisation for the next 30 years, moving to Winchester and its laboratory in Itchen Abbas in 1994, until I retired in 2013.

In the UK, there are four main groups of vets working for the government. By far the largest group are the VOs, who are based in animal health offices around the country and are responsible for implementing farm legislation surrounding TB controls, welfare and licensing requests. They are also a first point of contact if a suspect notifiable disease such as foot-and-mouth is reported. The second group are mainly office-based in central London and include the chief veterinary officer and his or her team responsible for developing the policies that are implemented in the field in consultation with wider organisations, including the European Union in particular. The third group are those involved in pure or applied research and they are located mainly in Weybridge. I worked for the fourth, undoubtedly elite, VIO group based in regional laboratories scattered throughout England and Wales.

The remit dictating our work was quite varied. The day-to-day job was to provide a laboratory, post-mortem and consultative service to farm animal/livestock units, not directly with each farm but through the farm's own vet. So I spent much of my time on the telephone to vets in practice discussing their problem cases, advising where I could, helping to devise laboratory testing protocols and then reporting results, often with further discussion. Carcasses of the full spectrum of farmed animals were brought in for post-mortem examination, from a day-old chick to an adult bovine. They also included zoological species that were closely related to our farm animals, including giraffes, four of which I eventually subjected to a full post-mortem (PM). We also went out on joint farm visits, usually with the farm's own vet to investigate severe or unusual cases in which we had a particular interest.

I have focused on the changes that have taken place during my life, and they are many and varied. Some have resulted in tangible improvements, but others perhaps have had the opposite effect. The changes that have occurred in the Veterinary Investigation (VI) service (now part of the Animal Health and Veterinary Laboratories Agency AHVLA) have been immense, and have been driven predominantly by the need to implement government financial targets placed on MAFF and Defra by the Treasury. Although all organisations have to change and adapt to current circumstances, it can be both difficult and at times frustrating to ensure that the service provided to customers and clients (essentially veterinary practitioners and farmers) and also ultimately to government itself does not deteriorate as a direct or indirect result.

When I first joined the organisation, it consisted of 24 laboratories (VI Centres) scattered strategically throughout England and Wales. After three major reviews over 30 years, the network has shrunk to only six AHVLA regional laboratories in England and Wales (and the poultry facility at Lasswade in Scotland) currently undertaking post-mortem examinations.

In 1983, it was essentially a free service; any vet or farmer could bring in a carcass or send in samples for testing without being charged. At that time the laboratory was busy with a constant flow of material being brought in – much of it unsuitable! When charging was introduced not long after I joined the organisation, we collectively held our breath, thinking it would signal the end of the service. In reality, it made very little difference, but did eliminate the 'rubbish' submissions, such as a long-dead rotten sheep! Most test prices have gradually increased to take into account the actual cost of undertaking each test, balanced against the demand for the test and its potential value to the farmer and veterinary surgeon. Many tests, however (such as the ELISA serology test) are actually cheaper as the technology has refined and automated the testing process.

So this does pose the question as to why the government appeared to be content to subsidise this service to farmers and essentially continue paying my salary for 30 years?

As a VIO, you are always aware you have three clients for whom you are working. The farm owners and their livestock are the end point customers – your service certainly benefits them. This work is carried out through the farm's own vet, thus the work that we do helps them to provide a better service to their clients through our undertaking of tests and PMs and interpreting results. The third customer is the government and, by inference, the general population. For 30 years, I have been undertaking surveillance work, mainly in the field of animal disease alongside the routine diagnostic work.

Our constant remit is to keep a watching brief for new and emerging threats. These have included recognising new diseases such as BSE, assessing the possibility of MRSA in farm animals, monitoring the incursion of exotic diseases into the

UK such as avian influenza, looking for any potential threat to the human food chain through chemical contamination or zoonotic diseases (those potentially transferred between animals and man) and looking into the welfare implications of new feeding and management systems.

In Carmarthen, I met another individual who had a major influence on my career – Gwyn Jones, who was the senior veterinary investigation officer at the Carmarthen laboratory. Peter Swire was the second VIO and I was to take over as the third. Our catchment area was the whole of south Wales, from Pembrokeshire in the west to the Severn Bridge in the east. There was another laboratory in Aberystwyth and one in Bangor, the three providing the service to Welsh agriculture that I hope was appreciated.

Gwyn suggested I shadow him initially, particularly in the post-mortem room. Although I had undertaken the occasional post-mortem while in practice, they were mainly at hunt kennels or knacker's yards, and most often on heaps of viscera left on the floor after the carcass had been opened. I had undertaken a fair few PMs on lambs while in Devon and as it was March and the lambing season was imminent, I could at least recognise some of the more common problems such as lamb dysentery and pulpy kidney (both now rare after 30 years and a successful vaccination programme), E. coli scour and septicaemia, and navel and joint ill.

There was no formal training in pathology, it was very much a case of learning on the job and I spent as much time as I could shadowing both Gwyn and Peter. Living on my own in a hotel in the early weeks also gave me the opportunity to revise my pathology notes and work my way through textbooks and any other laboratory information I could get my hands on. I began to enjoy the work as my confidence and knowledge began to grow, and learning new approaches, disease profiles and laboratory data became almost an obsession. The stimulus was always to be one step ahead of the veterinary practitioner who phoned for advice. To begin with, I did not hesitate to say I didn't know the information they wanted but that I would find out and let them know. Sometimes it was just a case of asking Gwyn or Peter but increasingly now I was building up my own knowledge base in my head. I began filing information away in paper format in a filing system, something that I added to for 30 years and still referred to on occasion up to my retirement. It was my 'living library'.

Shortly after I began to work in Carmarthen, I was sent on a two-week familiarisation course to learn about the activities, roles and responsibilities of the SVS. The first week was spent at the government veterinary headquarters at Tolworth, in Surrey. I was somewhat taken aback when I arrived on my first day to be directed to a disused army hospital on the edge of the main A3 road into central London which was surrounded by a barbed wire fence. The chief veterinary officer (CVO) and the rest of the hierarchy all had offices within this complex. The meat hygiene and import/export divisions were in the modern, high-rise building across the road that was referred to as Tolworth Tower, although they only occupied part of one floor.

There were nine of us in this new entrant group, including a future CVO, a future director of veterinary surveillance, a future eminent veterinary parasitologist and me. Although we had never met before, we got on well together and were advised to go across the road to a bowling alley called Charrington Bowl that served a good lunch. While there, we were surprised to see the CVO and other members of the veterinary hierarchy eating and holding informal lunchtime meetings in a booth. I often drive past this now derelict Tolworth site on my way along the A3 and my mind strays back to those early days as a ministry vet. As an aside, my mother used to refer to my new job as having joined the ministry, the Ministry of Agriculture, Fisheries and Food, or MAFF, as it was then. On more than one occasion, she had to explain that I had not taken holy orders and become a priest.

During our first week, we learned about the various roles and responsibilities of the different groups within SVS. These included those at the London headquarters who dealt mainly with the development and strategic implementation of UK government and EU legislation and the regional staff involved in its delivery. The work itself was broken down into a number of streams, such as animal welfare, notifiable disease, tuberculosis and import/export. There has been little change from then to the work streams of today.

During the second week, we moved to the Central Veterinary Laboratory at Weybridge to focus on the lab elements of the work and, more importantly for me, the area of work that interested me most. We moved through the various departments such as bacteriology, virology, pathology, parasitology, immunology and serology and met for the first time many of the eminent scientists who featured so regularly in scientific papers in the pages of the *Veterinary Record*, many of whom became close associates. Most of the time was spent getting to know how each department functioned and how they could have an impact on the work I was to carry out in the VI centres. This also enabled me to develop my network of contacts that was to grow over the next 30 years.

As part of this training period, we also spent one day at the Institute of Animal Health (now Pirbright Institute) in Pirbright, Surrey, which was, and still is, home to the World Reference Laboratory for Foot-and-Mouth Disease. I subsequently revisited on three occasions for refresher sessions and worked there for four months during the 2001 FMD outbreak. In addition to its role as the FMD reference laboratory, Pirbright also undertook research work (and still does today) on a number of other notifiable diseases that pose a threat to the UK and from which we maintain a freedom such as swine fever, African swine fever, swine vesicular disease, goat pox and rinderpest.

For our visit a number of trials had been set up, each of which culminated in a group of animals exhibiting clinical signs of these notifiable diseases that I had only previously read about or seen photographs of. It was important that I had experience of each condition as part of my job, as the next phase of my career was to provide a front-line defence against the potential incursion of these diseases into the UK, so I had to be able to recognise them. On the day of my first visit, I had the opportunity to examine cattle and pigs showing classical FMD lesions with large blistering areas on their tongues and around their feet. Sheep did not feature in the experiments at the time of my visit or in subsequent visits – and it was sheep that presented the biggest diagnostic challenge in 2001. As I was one of the laboratory-based new entrants, I had a first-hand opportunity to carry out post-mortem examinations on a heifer with rinderpest that showed the characteristic 'zebra striping' of its terminal large bowel, and pigs affected with both African and classical swine fever. Now, 30 years later, African swine fever is perceived to be an increasing threat to the UK and the risk of importing FMD is always with us. Rinderpest, however, was declared by the United Nations in June 2011 to have been eradicated globally, only the second disease after smallpox to have been given this status.

In discussion on the evening after our Pirbright visit, my group was unanimous in agreeing the day had been really useful, giving us the opportunity to gain experience (and at that stage in our careers, the confidence) to deal with suspect incidents of notifiable disease that we could be called out for in the future. There was also a genuine feeling of sadness at what we had seen. Each of the animals presented to us had been healthy in the weeks leading up to our visit, only to be infected with one of the horrible diseases that needed to be studied and with which we needed to become familiar. They were managed as well as the facilities allowed but, due to the risk of these devastating viruses escaping from Pirbright, they were all kept in high containment facilities which were often very barren in comparison to those seen on conventional farms. For example, there was no straw bedding as it was difficult to dispose of safely, and the animals spent their time lying on rubber mats. I'm pleased to say a raised awareness of environmental enrichment has seen a great improvement in the living conditions of such animals today.

The risk of spread of each of these agents, but in particular FMD, meant we had to undergo a strict entry and departure regime to ensure we did not enable the escape of viruses. We each had to strip off completely (there were separate changing rooms for males and females I hasten to add), then don paper underwear and disposable overalls and waterproofs on the way in. We then reversed the process on the way out, with a complete shower and hair washing routine supervised by Pirbright staff. We also had to sign a declaration that we would not be visiting any livestock enterprises or handling livestock for the next seven days as there was a slight risk we might have been carrying the FMD virus in our nasal chambers.

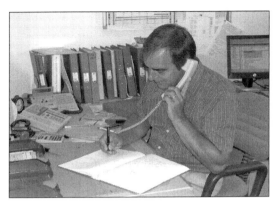

I spent many hours discussing cases with veterinary practice colleagues as a VIO (photo Winchester in 2008).

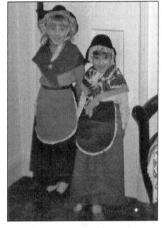

My daughters Maddy and Jess in their Welsh costumes and off to primary school on St David's day.

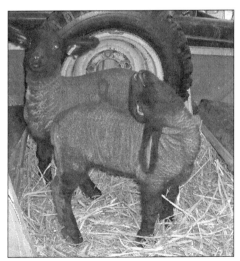

Case discussion with practising vets was an important part of the daily work of a VIO – the lamb in front shows a characteristic "tar-gazing" attitude, in this case caused by cerebrocortical necrosis (CCN).

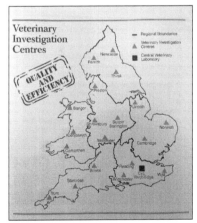

The network of laboratories when I joined the state veterinary service in 1983 – now only six.

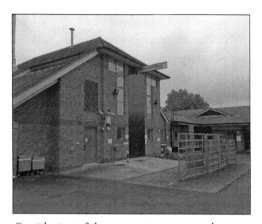

Outside view of the post-mortem room and handling race at Winchester Regional Laboratory.

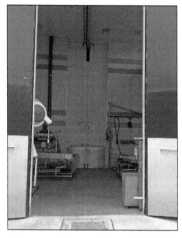

View into the post-mortem room at Winchester – tall doors enable large carcasses to be moved in via an overhead gantry.

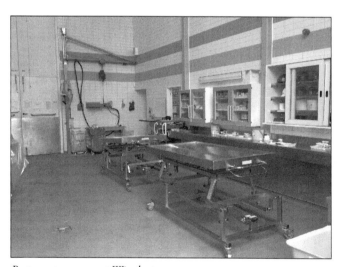

Post-mortem room at Winchester.

Chapter 12

Veterinary Detective Work on the Front Line

After my training period was completed, I returned to Carmarthen and got into the daily routine of case discussion with veterinary practitioners across south Wales on a consultancy basis (hence the constant need to be up to date). I also interpreted and reported on laboratory test results and undertook post-mortem examinations on a wide range of species. Carmarthen was a particularly busy post-mortem centre and I was able to rapidly build up my expertise. Conditions such as pulpy kidney, lamb dysentery, calf pneumonia and salmonella became almost a daily occurrence. By the time I eventually retired, there were hardly any of the diseases and other conditions affecting UK livestock that I had not experienced at first hand, often on many occasions.

The daily contact with veterinary practitioners across south Wales meant many became close friends. Being a civil service establishment, we had regular tea breaks at 10.30am, 12.30pm (for lunch) and 3.30pm, when we would gather in the tearoom unless we were busy. Our local vets were well aware of this and many would call in for a cup of tea while they were dropping off samples or if they were simply in the area. Our open door policy meant I had a regular stream of visiting vets calling in to discuss cases at first hand or results I had sent out. This was an extremely useful interchange of information. Vets were telling me about cases they were dealing with, trends they had identified and changes to farm management procedures they had experienced at the same time as I was hopefully helping them with their caseloads. Local vets and visiting farmers were often invited into the PM room to watch us carrying out the examination on their patients or livestock they owned. I felt part of the farming community in south Wales and genuinely believed I was carrying out the job that I felt I was being paid to do – namely supplying expert advice alongside a diagnostic laboratory and post-mortem service. At the same time, I was providing government with the grass roots surveillance information on the health and welfare of the UK livestock industry that it needed.

This was all to change over the intervening years, however, and increasingly a barrier was created between us and the veterinary practitioners. This was partly dictated by concerns over building and staff security (in the wake of terrorist activity directed at government buildings and staff) and partly by health and safety concerns. It began with all doors to the laboratory and PM room being locked – there was no longer an open door policy. All visitors had to ring a bell, be let into the building, sign a book, be given a visitor badge and escorted to whoever they wanted to meet. We received complaint after complaint from our practice 'friends', who while accepting that this had to be done, eventually and increasingly voted with their feet in that they called in, dropped off their samples, and left without speaking to anyone. I personally felt that this was a valuable loss of potential surveillance information and good-will, as although visits were often of a 'semi-social nature' (vet talking to vet), we did inevitably discuss cases, caseloads and other potentially useful topics. When I eventually moved to the newly refurbished laboratory in Winchester, these protocols were already firmly established, and I never really developed the close personal working relationships with the Winchester catchment area vets that I had enjoyed during my time in Carmarthen.

Health and safety has to be an important issue when dealing with potentially harmful pathogens, as we were doing on a daily basis. First and foremost, let me make it clear that I do not disagree with the need to have a firm policy in place. What I found increasingly frustrating was the number of rules and regulations being put in place by individuals, many of whom had not worked in the environment I had. I found myself constantly assessing my adherence to these, both consciously and subliminally – particularly in the post-mortem room itself. In Carmarthen in the late 1980s it was not unusual to have 20 individual submissions of aborted lambs sent in for post-mortem examination with a view to identifying likely infectious agents such as *Chlamydophila abortus* (the cause of enzootic abortion of ewes (EAE)), *Toxoplasma gondii*, or *Campylobacter* spp. These were all laid out around the post-mortem room, and we literally walked around examining and describing lesions in each one, taking whatever samples we needed to confirm a diagnosis. Although I had examined hundreds of such submissions in this 'relaxed manner', laboratory and post-mortem room health and safety policies began to be implemented and expanded to the point that I had to wear a full airstream helmet or carry out the procedure in a safety cabinet rather than on the bench as I had done previously. Before any sampling was undertaken, I had to prepare, stain and examine a smear from the placenta or foetus, looking specifically for *Coxiella burnettii*, the causative organism of a condition referred to as Q fever. Only when this condition had been cleared were we able to proceed with the sampling and testing protocol. Q fever has increasingly been recognised as an occupational risk, i.e. an organism that can be potentially hazardous to anyone working on material that may itself be contaminated with the causative organism. As with many health and safety policies that have been implemented across many of our daily activities, I did find this frustrating due to the increased amount of time spent on each submission. However, I fully supported the policy for both myself and those working with me (for whom I was responsible) in the post-mortem room environment.

Regularly, I allowed groups of students from agricultural colleges and sixth-formers hoping to gain entry to a vet school into the post-mortem room to experience the sights, sounds and smells first hand. It was always a popular part of the school visits that we developed progressively during my time in Winchester. Health and safety procedures also stopped this access and I had to describe how I did a PM using a PowerPoint presentation, something I felt particularly frustrated about. I genuinely felt that I had the knowledge and skills to ensure the safety of any student observing and surely the benefit must have outweighed the risk.

One such visit by a young farmers' club in Carmarthen at the time when I could take visitors into the post-mortem room did stick in my mind, but for a different reason. It was always my approach to outline to the visitors what we did, before heading for the laboratories, where we laid on some demonstrations, finishing in the post-mortem room. A number of the displays were fixed specimens in pots of formol saline. These were mainly roundworms, tapeworms and liver fluke, while other smaller parasites and bacteria were placed under a microscope for visitors to look at after being shown how to focus on the object. On this occasion, I had described what the young farmers should be seeing down each microscope, one specimen of which was of a *Psoroptes ovis* sheep scab mite. I had told them to pay particular attention to the shape of the mite in the centre of the image and described the leg structure and length that we used to differentiate it from other mange mites. One by one they looked down this microscope and one by one they all agreed they could see clearly what I had described. It wasn't until they were moving off from the area that I realised I had not turned the microscope on. All they could see was blackness but, as with the emperor's new clothes, no one dared admit it. In later years we had video cameras attached to microscopes which displayed images on to TV screens. These made my discussion much easier and relatively foolproof.

Another area that I became increasingly frustrated with was quality. Don't get me wrong, the quality of the work that my colleagues and I undertook had to be high class. However, the organisation did appear to lose its way in later years to the extent that quality appeared (at least to me) to become a higher priority than the efficient and rapid service I had always aspired to deliver to my practice colleagues and their livestock clients.

As an example, for many years I described in my reports on mastitic milk samples submitted for bacteriological examination the presence of *Staphylococcus aureus* (an important mastitis pathogen) the day following receipt. This was based on the morphological appearance of the isolate on the agar plate and on a stained smear under the microscope. This was coupled with the appearance of the milk on receipt and the accompanying history. In the later years of my time as a VIO, it could take up to three working days to undertake a range of confirmatory tests, only still to finish up calling it a 'likely' *Staphylococcus aureus*. In my view, this made it look as if we were still unsure.

Other labs such as UKAS (United Kingdom Accreditation Service) without the burden of a rigorous quality programme adopted by my organisation would not hesitate to call the organism by its designated name, without the word 'likely' and in a much shorter time. It came as no surprise that we increasingly became perceived as providing a slower and more expensive service and much of the routine diagnostic work was gradually lost. Our contact with practices and farm clients reduced as a result. Admittedly, as the service we provided was heavily subsidised by the government, the inevitable argument of unfair competition (highly specialised laboratories and facilities and subsidised test costs) often arose from our competitors and, with the need to cut the cost to the taxpayer, this perception became inevitable.

Having left practice with a 'have a go' attitude, it was pleasing to be allowed to follow this path at the Carmarthen laboratory and, in particular, with the local approach to dealing with sheep affected with gid. This is the colloquial term used to describe a condition more correctly referred to as coenuriasis, in which one or more parasitic cysts develop most commonly in the brain and occasionally in the spinal cord. *Coenurus cerebralis,* to give the cyst its correct name, is the intermediate host of the tapeworm *Taenia multiceps* that lives in the intestinal tract of mainly farm dogs and foxes. The tapeworm eggs are deposited on pasture in the dog or fox faeces and following faecal breakdown are taken in by grazing sheep. The parasite then passes through the body of the sheep, becoming eventually lodged in the brain or spinal cord, where it begins to grow. The resulting pressure causes the clinical signs of gid. If the sheep dies and is then scavenged and eaten by dogs or foxes, or if the head of a sheep that is culled either while affected while or incubating the disease is fed to the farm dogs (common practice at the time), then the life cycle continues.

The clinical signs displayed depend on the location and size of the cyst. If it is within the cerebral hemispheres then the sheep will tend to walk in circles deviating to the side in which the cyst is located. If it is in the cerebellum, the lesions are more severe and cause marked incoordination, often with the head deviated upwards and referred to as a star-gazer attitude.

Live suspect cases were admitted to the laboratory and kept in a small paddock outside my window. This was so I could observe them regularly without the obvious stress of me handling them in a strange place and away from other flock members, the company of which sheep will always crave. Once I had decided the sheep was affected with gid and I had a fair idea where the cyst was located, the animal was brought into the post-mortem room, given a thorough examination and then anaesthetised ready for surgery.

Gwyn had an interest in this procedure and taught me the basics; it was, to be blunt, very basic brain surgery. Once anaesthesia was complete, and with knowledge of the approximate location of the cyst, the head was shaved and prepared for surgery. Using a hand-held trephine after the skin was incised, a circular portion of skull bone was removed by a gentle sawing motion – the skull bone overlying the cyst was often softened due to the local pressure of the growth. As the bone was removed, it was hoped the cyst would be visible through the tough dura mater covering the brain and would begin to pop out as the dura was incised. If totally successful, the cyst could be encouraged to fall out of the brain tissue by turning the sheep's head upside down. The cyst wall was very thin and great care had to be taken not to burst it. The overall success rate was around 50 per cent, which does not sound too high. However, it does mean that half the sheep effectively coming in for a post-mortem examination were reprieved and sent home alive after successful surgery. The deal was the owner would be charged the full post-mortem rate regardless of whether the operation was a success or not. Some cases were confirmed by surgery, others by continuing to post-mortem if the cyst was deemed inoperable. Cerebellar and spinal column cysts were always the latter. It is amazing just how little of their cerebral cortex sheep actually need to lead a full and healthy life. These were very much the good old days of the VI service that I am pleased to have experienced.

One of Peter Swire's interests was liver fluke and he, together with the parasitology department at the Central Veterinary Laboratory in Weybridge, provided a regular forecast on the likely prevalence of this devastating parasite. Parasites and their life cycles have always interested me from my first lectures at the RVC.

Liver fluke, as outlined earlier, is a parasite of the liver that affects ruminants in the UK. The mature parasite lives in the gall bladder and bile ducts of the liver. It lays eggs, which pass out via the bile into the gut to be deposited on the pasture in faeces. The eggs hatch and then need to find and attack a small mud snail, passing through it to be deposited back on the pasture as cercaria. This is a developmental stage of the liver fluke that following encystment is taken in again by ruminants grazing in the area. This stage then penetrates the gut wall and the liver capsule to complete the life cycle.

Knowing the various environmental requirements of the life cycle enables us to predict the likely impact – higher in wet areas and wet climates that favour the mud snail and lower in dry areas and following long dry spells. Under Peter's direction, the Carmarthen staff including myself would visit areas where the snail habitat was well known. Using a wire grid thrown randomly on to a patch of wet pasture we would then get on our hands and knees and count and collect the number of snails we could see within the confines of the grid. This was carried out in several other locations, arriving at an average count to be compared with other visits to the same area. Some snails were returned to the laboratory and kept alive in an aquarium, while others were dissected under a microscope where we looked for the redia, the parasite intermediate stage found in the snail liver.

All our local west Wales information was submitted to Weybridge and collated to produce a national fluke forecast. Not surprisingly, this approach did not continue and in fact the parasitology department in Weybridge was eventually disbanded, much to our collective dismay. Any further forecasting was to be carried out by the industry and in particular the pharmaceutical companies responsible for the manufacture and distribution of the flukicide products.

You could argue the primary reason I was paid a salary as a civil servant during my time as a government vet was to provide surveillance information on new and emerging diseases – BSE was a prime example – note changes and trends in known diseases and make an early identification of exotic notifiable diseases. I feel I played my part in all these areas. From day one, I was encouraged to pursue anything that sounded unusual, of widespread distribution or genuinely interesting, and to provide follow-up examination free of charge (to encourage submissions) or to undertake farm visits with the farm's vet. We were also encouraged to publish these findings in the scientific press for the benefit of others and by the time I retired I had published in excess of 100 papers.

My first publication in the pages of the *Veterinary Record* was one that is still often quoted and referred to today, and also ignited my interest in ruminant diseases associated with *Clostridia* spp. Shortly after I began working in Carmarthen, I had a series of adult cows sent in for post-mortem examination, each of which had died from a severe gas-gangrenous infection of the upper hind limb (rump) musculature from which we identified differing *Clostridium* species using fluorescent antibody tests (FATs). The condition was referred to as a clostridial myositis, or more colloquially as malignant oedema. It is linked with the proliferation of bacteria deep in the muscle tissue and often follows a deep penetrating wound.

My interest ignited, I began following up these cases, which occurred on more than one farm in the time frame of my study, with the submitting practitioners. It transpired that each animal had received an injection of a prostaglandin product used for controlling the oestrus cycle. Other similar cases followed over the next few months and these included injections of vitamin products and of a wormer preparation. As each case involved a pharmaceutical product they were all reported to the Veterinary Medicines Directorate as suspect adverse reactions to licensed products so the manufacturers could undertake their own investigations. I wrote the series up in a paper accepted as a short communication to the *Veterinary Record* in 1984 entitled *Apparent Iatrogenic Clostridial Myositis in Cattle*, the word 'iatrogenic' referring to any condition actually caused by the intervention of a veterinary surgeon or physician.

I continued to develop an interest in these diseases, writing a number of refresher articles for the BCVA, the *UK Vet* journal and the lay farming press. I was eventually deemed the AHVLA clostridial disease consultant and, as a result, I was invited by a manufacturer to speak at the launch of its new multi-valent clostridial vaccine known as Covexin10 in the UK, Holland, Belgium and Italy.

It was the variety of cases that came through the laboratory that I found most fascinating. I had enjoyed my time in practice immensely but there were many occasions when I was left asking questions about why an animal had died or what it was suffering from that I wasn't always able to answer. That was, unless I asked the farm to pay for a post-mortem or for laboratory tests that they often simply had no interest in. Working in a laboratory environment, however, meant I could pursue the cases that came my way in great detail, consulting with in-house experts if necessary. I rarely felt I had no idea what the problem was, though, and this gave me great job satisfaction.

As a simple example, I received a phone call while in Carmarthen from a practitioner who wished to send in some ducklings that had developed misshapen beaks and feet. They were not long hatched and the beaks were becoming twisted and there were some raw lesions developing on the feet. There were also some fresh lesions resembling blisters. It was also apparent that only the ducklings with white beaks and feet were afflicted, those with coloured beaks and feet seeming to be unaffected. I had never seen this previously but it did resemble a condition I was familiar with in cattle referred to as 'photosensitisation' in which the white skin of cattle can become severely damaged when they have been exposed to certain poisonous plants such as St John's wort that contain photodynamic agents that become activated in the skin by sunlight. The pigmented skin is unaffected. These ducklings had to be affected with something similar.

On questioning the owners, it transpired they had moved the ducklings and their mother to a new enclosed area which had long grass and weeds that had been strimmed. I asked them to return with any plants that were still growing undisturbed and they came back with several including giant hogweed (*Heracleum mantegazzianum*), a plant I discovered subsequently does contain sap that is activated on skin when exposed to sunlight. I assumed the pigment had protected the sensitive beak and feet of the unaffected ducklings. I contacted a friend who was a consultant dermatologist in the local Glangwili General Hospital and he confirmed that he saw cases of severe blistering on the exposed arms and legs of strimmer operators who cut through the stems of giant hogweed. This liberated the sap on to their skin and it then became activated by sunlight exposure. He had also seen similar lesions around the mouths of children who had used the stem of this tall plant as pea shooters. This was an ideal letter to send to the *Veterinary Record* to warn vets of this potential risk.

One of the more serious incidents I first investigated and reported on was a severe pneumonia and pleurisy syndrome that was killing adult cattle very quickly. The first case I saw was sent in to us on the afternoon of our laboratory Christmas lunch, arriving while we were still seated and finishing the meal in a local pub. A phone call summoned me back to the post-mortem room where a well-grown Holstein Friesian cow was hanging on the hoist. I had spoken to the practitioner and had received some background, although this was fairly minimal. The cow was milking well but suddenly developed a temperature, stopped eating, began breathing very heavily and was in increasing distress until it died. Antibiotic treatment had done very little.

At post-mortem examination, the thoracic cavity contained a large quantity of clear fluid and both lungs showed a very severe fulminating pneumonia, with thick pleural deposits over the lung tissue so the lung lobes were sticking together. The lung tissue itself was solid throughout – around 70 per cent of the total volume – so no wonder there had been such severe respiratory distress when alive. Quite significantly within this tissue were focal areas of severe lung necrosis. The presentation was identical to that seen in one of our notifiable diseases known as contagious bovine pleuropneumonia (CBPP), a condition we still do not have in the UK and which is confined currently mainly to Africa. I had no choice but to report my suspicion to veterinary colleagues in the animal health office nearby. They visited the farm, examined the remaining cattle for signs of illness and investigated possible movements on to the site.

In the meantime, I contacted Weybridge and arranged for tissue and blood samples from the cow to be delivered overnight. I also made arrangements for laboratory staff in the mycoplasma section to be prepared to receive and process my samples. The causative organism of CBPP is *Mycoplasma mycoides* and this required specialist laboratory input. We also set up our own cultures in Carmarthen. The following day we had heavy pure growths of an organism at that time referred to as *Pasteurella haemolytica,* now renamed as *Mannheimia haemolytica.* This is an organism well known to me as a cause of pneumonia in sheep and as a secondary invader in calf pneumonia, but not a known cause of such severe disease in adult cattle in the UK. There was also some similarity to a condition referred to as 'shipping' or 'transit' fever in the USA but, as the name suggests, it tended to occur in animals stressed as a result of recent transportation and my case had no such history. All tests for CBPP came back negative and we decided it was probably a one-off.

Over the next few weeks, however, we had a number of other almost identical cases that occurred on the same farm and others, and cases were also reported at another VI centre in Langford. We undoubtedly had a new and emerging condition here. We could categorise the clinical presentation and the pathology, and had confirmed consistently that *Mannheimia haemolytica* was the main causative agent. On each occasion we ruled out CBPP. Our main question was why were these cases occurring? What was the trigger?

We did identify other possible contributing organisms such as IBR (infectious bovine rhinotracheitis), a respiratory virus of cattle, and *Mycoplasma bovis,* an organism most commonly associated with calf pneumonia, but neither organism was a consistent presence. We compared Met Office data and there did seem to be some correlation between sudden changes in weather conditions from warm to very cold, dry to humid or cold to warm, but we really had no idea why these cases began to develop. I presented our findings at the next meeting of the BCVA. I also received an invitation to speak on the same subject at the World Buiatrics (Cattle Medicine) congress in Edinburgh in 1994, in front of an audience of around 1,250 – my largest ever. The condition has ebbed and flowed ever since and is reported sporadically by practitioners and VI centres at other locations within the UK, often quoting my original texts. We still do not know the full reason why this disease develops.

In the late spring of 1997, I was presented with a severe lameness problem in a Sussex sheep flock that I did not realise at the time was the world's first recorded case of a condition now referred to as contagious ovine digital dermatitis (CODD). I was asked to visit the flock by the local veterinary practice, which was concerned at the number of cases of severe lameness it was being asked to examine.

When I arrived into the main lambing area (it was the height of the lambing season) it was apparent we were dealing with a serious problem. There were recumbent sheep all around the pen, many of which were making an effort to get to their feet and hobble away, while others tried but failed. There were many hungry lambs around the pen because they simply could not get at the udders of ewes unable to rise. As a result lamb mortality that year was much higher than average. Several ewes had already been destroyed on humane grounds and I had to advise that others should be similarly culled. I had seen many lame sheep during my time as a veterinary surgeon and was very familiar with the condition referred to as footrot, a particularly virulent and infectious foot condition caused by two anaerobic organisms, of which *Dichelobacter nodosus* is considered to be the primary pathogen. There were similarities between footrot and what I was presented with, but this was much more severe. Many of the ewes were infected in two and occasionally three feet. Many claws had been completely 'shelled off', exposing the delicate soft laminar tissue beneath and making walking extremely painful. This may happen in footrot cases but is rare. The damage to the claw in footrot tends to work from the sole upwards, separating the wall from the underlying laminae but not detaching it completely. These cases appeared to be more active at the junction between skin and horn at the top of the claw and this resulted in a weakening of the attachment and eventual loss of the claw.

To further confound my diagnosis, the flock was well managed. The feet were in good condition with no obvious overgrowth, and the sheep were on clean bedding and had been vaccinated against footrot. I took foot swabs and portions of cast-off horn for bacteriological examination and returned to the laboratory. Our failure to grow *Dichelobacter nodosus* also tended to rule out classic footrot. In my mind, I was dealing not with a new disease but with a different manifestation of an existing condition and I coined the title acute virulent footrot.

I immediately prepared a letter to send to the *Veterinary Record* written in collaboration with the practitioner who had first invited me on to the farm. We described what we had seen, asking specifically if other practitioners had encountered anything similar. Additional, more specialist, laboratory testing using scanning electron microscopy and lesion histopathology identified *spirochaete* organisms similar to those identified in lesions of digital dermatitis, another more recently identified disease of the feet of cattle. By this time, we knew that this was definitely not footrot and the general feeling was that, as the aetiology was similar to digital dermatitis of cattle (although the pathology was quite different), the condition would be termed contagious ovine digital dermatitis (CODD). My original letter and a subsequent follow-up letter are still quoted as describing the first case of this condition. This is, I believe, one of the best examples of my involvement in a new and emerging disease investigation during my time in Carmarthen and Winchester.

In an earlier chapter I described my attempts at undertaking a rumenotomy while looking for fragments of metal that had been swallowed and finished up in the reticulum, the second stomach of the cow that lies near the diaphragm. Metallic fragments can penetrate the reticular wall as it contracts cyclically and they eventually pass through the diaphragm and into the chest cavity, often finishing up in the heart.

It was during my time in Winchester that we began to notice a change in the pattern of this disease and in particular the presenting signs. Traditionally, the condition could be identified by standing on the left of the cow and applying increasing upward pressure with fist and knee into the area just behind the ribcage on the lower abdominal wall. This action would cause the cow to grunt with pain if there was damage to the area due to a penetrating foreign body. The alternative was to pinch the withers of the cow, just behind its shoulders. This in turn would cause the cow to dip, literally stretching the ventral abdominal wall area and again causing the cow to grunt. These new cases were showing no such signs, yet we were finding that the reticular wall had been penetrated at post-mortem and we were also finding very sharp thin bits of wire that were causing the problem. These were identified as fragments of the radial steel found in car tyres and yet again we were looking at a new and emerging problem.

Tyres were used to hold down the sheeting on silage clamps to keep them airtight and could often be seen from the road as one drove past. Previously, any farmer could turn up at their local tyre depot and fill the trailer with old worn tyres to replace any that were disintegrating on the clamp. A change to the EU waste legislation in the early 1990s, however, meant that tyres had to be disposed of in a structured way, so they were no longer available to the general public in this way. That resulted in the existing tyres beginning to disintegrate badly, resulting in fragments of wire dropping into the silage being fed to cattle. It was these fragments we were finding at post-mortem. This change also coincided with an increase in feeding a total mixed ration (TMR) to dairy cows, whereby the ration constituents, including silage, were combined in a trailer that chopped and mixed the constituents together, before dispensing the final mix in front of the cattle. Tyres or tyre fragments were often inadvertently chopped and mixed with the final ration.

We began an awareness campaign in the veterinary and farming press highlighting these dangers, encouraging farms to carry out a tyre audit before making the next season's silage, to ensure that no tyres were badly worn. Many farms resorted to mass medication of all cows at risk with a magnet. This was given by mouth and would drop into the reticulum so pieces of metal would be attracted and hopefully not pass through the wall and cause the condition that is more correctly referred to as traumatic reticulopericarditis. I co-wrote an article for the veterinary profession on this subject highlighting its recognition and prevention in a journal titled *In Practice,* a supplement to the *Veterinary Record.* Other methods of holding the sheeting down on to the surface of silage clamps have now been identified and the condition is seen far less frequently, hopefully in part as a result of my involvement.

I have always been fascinated with these new and emerging diseases and was involved in many during my time working as a VIO. I remember being called to investigate a series of cases of a condition in calves that was referred to originally as blood sweating disease or later as the bleeding calf syndrome. These were two excellent descriptions, each capturing in a nutshell exactly how each condition presented. It affected young calves in the first one to three weeks of life. One of the first signs reported by farmers and private vets were small rivulets of blood running down the legs and body surface, so the affected animal appeared to be sweating blood. These same calves also bled easily from any injection site and from the insertion site of an identification ear tag. Some also dripped blood from their noses and one dead calf I examined had blood in its tears. At post-mortem examination there were haemorrhages throughout the body, with large clots of blood filling the small intestine in some cases.

This was undoubtedly a new, emerging and very dramatic and unusual disease. As in all such cases, a multi-discipline approach was quickly rolled out that defined the exact pathology, arrived at a case definition and then completed extensive questionnaire information from each case to identify possible common factors. The underlying cause was complex and did involve a particular cattle vaccine that had been administered to the dam (mother) of the affected calf, but this was only part of the story, as many million doses of this same vaccine had been used throughout Europe. Cases were only sporadic and quickly disappeared as the vaccine was initially removed from the market and then eventually modified and re-launched. I described the initial names given to the condition, blood sweating disease and bleeding calf syndrome, as being particularly accurate and descriptive of the condition, but although the terms are still used colloquially, the condition has now been renamed. In view of the defined pathology causing the condition, essentially a bone marrow disorder, it is now referred to as bovine neonatal pancytopenia (with the rather unfortunate acronym BNP). This condition will undoubtedly run its course and may never be seen again, a feature of a number of these new and emerging problems.

I have already described one investigation while I was working in Carmarthen that led me to suspect an exotic notifiable disease incursion (CBPP) which was ruled out very quickly. Several years later in Winchester I was faced with another similar scenario that began with the submission of four dead weaner pigs on a Friday afternoon. They were covered in haemorrhages under the skin surface, giving each one a very mottled appearance. I had to consider classical swine fever (CSF) as a likely cause and immediately contacted the local animal health office, which despatched a veterinary officer to the farm that same afternoon. As I continued with the post-mortem, I identified more and more lesions that I considered typical of CSF, including haemorrhages in the tonsils, bladder wall and over the surface of the kidney (so called turkey egg kidney – a classic CSF lesion), with multiple haemorrhages throughout other viscera.

This looked serious and, in discussion with the SVS headquarters in London, the farm was put under restriction and samples were rushed to Pirbright for CSF virology testing. These test results came back negative, much to everyone's relief, but we now had a conundrum. These pigs were presenting with pathology wholly consistent with that seen in CSF cases (and possibly even more convincing) yet the disease had been ruled out. As the farm was still losing pigs, on direct instruction from the CVO a team of us was despatched there to further investigate the case, but in particular to undertake more post-mortem examinations to build up a complete pathology profile. Over the next two days, the farm's own vet, an eminent pig pathologist called Stan Done, and I undertook around 50 post-mortem examinations and took many photographs and samples.

What we had been presented with on this occasion was not notifiable exotic disease, but another new and emerging disease of pigs in the UK now referred to as PMWS (postweaning multisystemic wasting syndrome). This is a circovirus infection acting in tandem with another newly recognised condition of pigs known as PDNS (porcine dermatitis and nephropathy syndrome). So on this occasion we thought we were dealing with a notifiable disease but, in fact, we were dealing with two recently identified conditions acting synergistically, wherein the end result is a more serious disease than the combination of the two would be expected to produce. This was again written up in the *Veterinary Record* for wider knowledge distribution and is still considered a primary differential diagnosis for CSF.

Over the years, I have been presented with some pretty unusual requests for help and input, none more unusual than ostriches in Swansea. Unbeknown to me at the time, a warehouse next to an MFI store on an industrial estate in Swansea was being used as a European quarantine station for ostriches being transported from Namibia to Canada. I was asked if I would attend to carry out some health checks and take some blood samples and ocular swabs as some of the birds had discharging eyes. Under normal circumstances, the local animal health office would have asked a local veterinary practitioner to undertake this work – but as no practitioner was available or willing to commit – I was asked by the local Divisional Veterinary Officer at the time to assume responsibility. I had never handled ostriches but was told the staff were skilled. So I turned up and walked into a surreal situation with around 50 adult ostriches, each reportedly worth several thousand pounds.

I had found out some information about ostriches before I left the office, so was aware they have a much better developed right than left jugular – leading to the myth that they only have one. What I hadn't prepared for were the problems related to handling these animals or even being anywhere near them. They stand more than 6 ft tall and are incredibly inquisitive – they will peck at anything that interests them such as spectacles, a pen in your pocket or your 'yurs', as my very Welsh assistant told me. I quickly found this out by a painful tug to what became a very red ear. They can also kick hard, so the standard protective gear was a hard hat and a cricket box. The manager of the unit had constructed a race area where the ostriches were walked in one by one. He then rolled a sock over his arm, grabbed the bird's head and rolled the sock over it, covering completely its eyes. The ostrich immediately became calm and I could then get on and examine and bleed it. I'm not sure if this behaviour is related to the stories of ostriches burying their heads in the sand but my patients were certainly oblivious to their surroundings. I suspect very few shoppers at the stores on this site were aware of what was going on in the warehouse, whose occupants all arrived in the early hours of the morning when no one was around.

I also visited a snail farm (yes, a snail farm) in mid Wales to investigate a problem of ill thrift in Giant African land snails. This alternative farm enterprise had contacted its local vet for help and advice and, as was so often the case with an unusual problem, had been referred to us. On arrival, I was taken out to a wooden shed with heat lamps and I walked in to be surrounded by these snails, grown for the gourmet market. They were on the walls, the floor and the roof – everywhere. I took some details of feeding and any recent changes to understand their management, as any snail novice would. We decided I would take some back for post-mortem examination. This immediately presented me with a problem – how should I kill them humanely? Rightly or wrongly, and to preserve the tissue I needed, I decided to place them in a deep freeze as I couldn't use any of the euthanasia approaches I normally adopted. After they were thawed out, I dissected each one and, to my surprise, actually got a diagnosis. They were heavily infested with nematode worms – this was why they were not growing.

We devised a worm control treatment and the weight gains recorded previously returned, much to mine and the owner's satisfaction.

It was while I was in Carmarthen that I had first-hand experience of what was a local natural disaster, namely flooding. In October 1987, the town suffered severe flooding when water from the river Towy burst its banks and left the Pensarn area under 12 ft of water. It was reportedly the result of a combination of factors including heavy recent rain, a high autumn tide and the release of water from the Llyn Brianne dam further upriver. Our car was having body repair work undertaken in Pensarn and was ready to be collected but we couldn't make it due to the flooding. It was moved in anticipation from the workshop, which reportedly ended up under 12 ft of water, to higher, supposedly safe ground, but even that was awash under 4 ft. I could see where my car was parked on *News at Ten* but could not see the vehicle until the following day when the flood water had receded and I could just see the top! Clearly, the car was a write-off.

We were down in Pensarn two days later collecting items from the car when a large group of people began walking towards us. We hadn't realised that Prince Charles and Princess Diana were touring the area, with massive media coverage. It was reportedly the first time they had been seen in public together for more than a month and after the visit they apparently again went their separate ways.

The flooding at that time and on other occasions resulted in a number of incidents of water dropwort poisoning in cattle. As the name suggests, this plant grows around water and if the river bank is undermined due to fast-flowing flood water, the plant is often uprooted and deposited on pasture as the water recedes. The roots of this plant resemble dahlia tubers and are referred to colloquially as dead men's fingers. They are highly attractive to grazing livestock, but are also highly toxic and can kill quickly. Most affected cattle are found dead. A diagnosis is made partly as a result of finding tubers on the pasture but also fragments in the rumen content.

Examination of such content was never my most enjoyable task but it did often yield a variety of plant fragments that needed to be identified. In such cases I could call on my childhood love of wild flower collecting and pressing, my poisonous plants lectures and practicals while at the RVC and my love of gardening to combine to help me with identification. Some were easy. The most common cause of sudden death plant poisoning in the UK is yew (*Taxus baccata*) and leaf and stem fragments were readily identifiable as the animal (usually cattle) died very quickly, before the leaf fragments could begin to be digested. Yew trees are commonly found in churchyards in the UK and many such incidents were seen in cattle in neighbouring fields, either when high winds blew down trees or branch debris into the cattle field or where tree clippings were thrown over the hedge or wall. One such yew poisoning case in which four steers died resulted from them gaining access to a hide built of yew branches in the corner of a field. Poachers had been shooting pheasants over the weekend from their shelter before leaving it for the ever inquisitive cattle to eat.

Oak (*Quercus robur*) trees are also very common throughout the UK and pose no problem to grazing livestock unless there is a particularly heavy fall of acorns. These acorns, if eaten in large quantities, can cause severe illness and death in grazing ruminants. Horses and pigs can eat acorns with few if any clinical signs. In the rumen of cattle and sheep in particular, the acorns release tannic acid which is broken down by rumen microbes into a product known as pyrogallol. This is a nephrotoxin, i.e. it causes kidney damage.

I investigated a number of cases in both Carmarthen and Winchester, all in sheep and cattle in years of heavy cropping. Some were found dead, others profoundly sick with diarrhoea. Post-mortem examination of those found dead and blood sampling of live affected animals confirmed kidney failure. What we realised in Carmarthen when the condition was beginning to be more recognised was that cattle in particular became 'addicted' to acorns, spending their entire time searching for them on the ground and even looking up into the trees for the next one to fall. We devised a simple test to check for this addiction by walking into the field with a bag or bucket of feed. The cattle and sheep that ran up to the feed on offer were not addicted and we could turn our attention to those hanging around the oaks. These could then be bled to check their kidney function and moved away from the acorns to recover. Sadly, dialysis is not on offer for farm animals, so any with compromised kidneys were often slaughtered on humane grounds. This is a prime example of how veterinary science and good farm stockmanship can combine forces.

One other plant that produced very dramatic signs in goats and sheep in particular is rhododendron. If the plant is eaten inadvertently the classic sign described is projectile vomiting, an extremely unusual presentation in ruminants. What actually occurs is the forceful expulsion of rumen content through the mouth and nose due to the presence of a plant toxin known as a vomitotoxin that acts on the vomiting centre in the brain, causing this uncontrolled regurgitation. It can kill and even those that survive this initial assault remain at risk from aspiration pneumonia if they inadvertently inhale the rumen content into their airways. The advice was always to cover them with an antibiotic course 'just in case'.

I maintained my interest in lameness, particularly in cattle, throughout my time in the state veterinary service. This was most likely as a legacy from my practice days when lame cows were dealt with on a daily basis. My involvement as a VIO usually saw me going out on joint farm visits with inexperienced practitioners presented not with individual cases but with either sudden outbreaks or escalating problems. Lameness in cattle is a truly multi-factorial disease, with nutrition, flooring materials, bedding availability and quality, cubicle and general housing layout all contributing. Each aspect needed to be assessed and amended where possible. I was also called on to examine abattoir specimens of feet or limbs removed and seized as part of a welfare infringement investigation. This was essentially forensic work, in which I developed an increasing expertise and interest. I managed the animal welfare programme of work across the laboratory network and became skilled in forensic examination and expert witness work in animal welfare prosecution cases brought by Defra or the RSPCA.

Every consumer of any food product purchased in the UK has the right to expect the product to be fresh, wholesome and free of any infectious agents or chemical and other residues. Another aspect of the work of a VIO was to investigate any incident in which the consumer might be put at risk and such investigations could be particularly vexing. By far the most common contaminant identified was lead and I investigated many such cases at both Carmarthen and Winchester.

Lead poisoning is seen most commonly in cattle, although any farmed species is potentially susceptible, including poultry. The most common clinical sign encountered is sudden death, whereby an animal is fit and well one day and found dead the next. After anthrax is ruled out in cattle (and this testing is routinely undertaken on all unexpected sudden death cases), then lead poisoning is always a strong candidate as a likely cause. Lead poisoning is confirmed by the demonstration of abnormally high levels of lead in the kidney or liver, where it tends to concentrate. If alive, the most common sign is blindness and other non-specific neurological signs that may include hyperexcitability at one end of the spectrum or immobility at the other. In these cases the diagnosis is made from demonstrating high levels of lead in the blood.

Animals found dead will never enter the food chain but live affected animals and others that may have taken a lower dose yet remain fit and healthy could potentially be slaughtered or their milk sold for human consumption. It is the liver and kidneys (the lead storage sites) that pose the greatest risk. Once lead poisoning is confirmed, the animals at risk are retained on the farm for a minimum of 90 days after the lead source is removed from their environment.

After the initial diagnosis is made, the farm is usually visited and the detective work then continues to identify a likely source. Lead has been slowly removed from our modern environment and we now have lead-free petrol, lead-free paint and the removal and replacement of old lead water pipes. It is not surprising, therefore, that the majority of sources of lead encountered were often historical in origin.

The cases I was involved with were many and varied and included calves having access to old flaking lead paint on doors used as temporary barriers in their pens, which they readily licked off, and cows licking ash around the margins of a bonfire on which timber coated with old lead paint had been burnt. One memorable case in which a number of heifers died resulted from them gaining access to an old rubbish tip after a tree growing over it had been blown down in the wind. The tip contained disintegrating tins of now solid, high lead content paint and this proved attractive to the inquisitive cattle, with one chunk even containing teeth marks.

Dumped car batteries still contain high levels of lead but cattle are normally protected from harm by the robust outer case. Electric fencing around the margins of fields is often powered by these batteries and they remain safe unless inadvertently driven over and crushed or thrown on to a bonfire, when the lead cell material becomes exposed. In one battery incident I was involved in while working in Winchester, some local boy racers had a habit of stealing cars and racing them around any field with an open gate before torching them for fun. On one such occasion, three cars had suffered this fate and were lying around a small coppice in the centre of a field. The farmer was not aware of their presence and he turned cattle into the field to graze. In this case, the battery had melted in the heat of the fire and the lead part of the cells was exposed. Heavy rain had created a surface covering of lead salts and cattle have a strong liking for a salty taste, often licking cars in winter as a result of a covering of road salt. Four well grown heifers died from acute lead poisoning as a result.

One more unusual chemical poisoning incident I became involved with was caused by metaldehyde, which is found in slug pellets. I received a phone call from a veterinary surgeon near the Winchester laboratory who said that a dairy cow had just been found dead on a nearby farm and several other cows were wandering around in a 'drunken state'. I undertook the post-mortem examination in the early afternoon and was presented with a cow obviously in good condition and with an udder full of milk. There were no lesions in any of the organs examined and I then moved on to the next part of my routine with a cow. This involved sifting through its rumen content to look for poisonous plants or anything else that could be toxic. As I separated the rumen content by hand, I could see small blue specks of between 3 and 5 mm in diameter. As I was a keen gardener, I recognised that these resembled the size and colour of slug pellets. Armed with this information, I arranged to head out to the farm later that afternoon to meet the vet who had phoned me and to confirm my suspicions.

It transpired that the owner had lit a bonfire in the corner of the field where the cows were grazing and, being inquisitive, they came up to see what was happening. Cows also seem to be attracted by smoke in summertime, possibly to help rid themselves of flies. The owner was using an old oil drum as an incinerator to burn mainly paper bags and scattered all around the incinerator were slug pellets, which were undoubtedly the source of the discolouration in the rumen content. Many of the bags had previously contained the pellets and as he screwed up each bag before placing it in the incinerator, the residual pellets had fallen on to the floor and became available to the cattle. The other affected cattle soon recovered and as none of them were destined for slaughter, restrictions were only placed on the milk from the whole herd. This was disposed of for four successive milkings before being deemed fit for human consumption again.

The proximity of Marwell Zoo and other zoological collections in south-east England meant that during my time in Winchester I was able to undertake a number of PM examinations on a wide range of species including three giraffes, an adult male lion, an adult tiger, wallabies, snakes and a wide variety of antelopes and birds. One of the giraffes, a male, died as a result of a ruptured bladder caused by a small bladder stone getting trapped in the urethra within its penis. It was very sad that such a small stone, less than 1 cm in diameter, could have killed such a magnificent creature. Both the adult lion and tiger died as a result of chronic interstitial nephritis – a relatively common problem in elderly domestic cats. We were also screening the brains of any big cat that died for evidence of FSE, or feline spongiform encephalitis, a number of cases of which were identified in domestic cats in the UK. Much of the meat fed to these big cats originated from 'fallen cattle', i.e. those that had died on a farm and had been taken to either a local knacker's yard or hunt kennels. It seemed likely the source of the FSE we saw in the big cats was the result of them eating dead cattle infected with BSE.

I have been involved in a number of unusual and quite bizarre investigations but none more so than the so-called Beast of Brechfa. I was asked while in Carmarthen to examine a dog that had been attacked and mauled by something near the village of Brechfa. It was a most unusual post-mortem since this dog, a collie type, had major injuries with penetrating bite wounds, but more significantly its spinal cord had been crushed. Whatever had attacked it was large and strong. My primary concern at that time was the potential risk such an animal, in my mind a rogue, very large dog, might pose to the public. So I contacted the police, who came to view my findings, and it wasn't long before the name the Beast of Brechfa was coined as word got around about what I had found.

The Welsh language TV channel S4C then sent a film crew to interview me. They were slightly irritated that I was English and could not speak Welsh but nevertheless the interview took place in our post-mortem room. I turned on the TV that night to view my performance and have to admit to having a wry smile as my voice had been dubbed into Welsh with a very strange high-pitched voice and my words were shown as English subtitles. They also interviewed a local man who had seen what he was convinced was a black panther jumping over a church wall. I have an open mind as to whether or not these mystery beasts exist. There have been a number of reported sightings around the UK, including the beast of Bodmin Moor and, of course, the Loch Ness monster.

During another TV appearance for the BBC Wales *Farming* programme, I had been asked to meet the crew at a farm near Aberystwyth to discuss the treatment and control of calf pneumonia. We were looking at the building design and ventilation, the stocking rates (essentially whether they were overcrowded or not) and some sick calves. All was going well until during one filming session, a low-flying jet came screaming over just above the building and simultaneously my interviewer, the camera and microphone team and myself all ducked as it was so loud. Playing the recording back later, however, we realised that although we were all startled, the cattle in the building barely flinched and carried on eating.

It did change my mind about one other more unusual issue I became involved with, namely claims against the Welsh government for losses related to cattle abortion resulting from low-flying aircraft. A proportion of cows will lose their calf during pregnancy simply due to genetic or physiological factors and akin to the small proportion of women who sadly suffer a miscarriage during pregnancy. Admittedly there are some infectious agents that will cause cows to abort, such as *Salmonella* spp. *Neospora caninum* and BVD virus, and in most instances infection with these agents will cause a series of abortions, not sporadic losses.

Farmers have claimed successfully that these sporadic abortions are due to low-flying aircraft startling the cows as they fly past. If material submitted to us to test for infectious agents ultimately found nothing and if it could be proven that planes were active in the vicinity of the abortion then the Welsh government had been paying compensation. Realising it was probably paying out too frequently, we were asked to be far more rigid in our approach by ruling out as many other causes as we could. We also requested where possible that the farm noted the times and trajectory of any planes nearby, even taking their identification marks if they were flying low enough for them to be seen. We carried on paying out for these, but from watching how little attention the calves during my BBC interview paid to the plane that sent us all reeling, it is hard to accept that cows can be stressed enough to abort. As an aside, I have wondered for years if any clip of us remains as it would be good enough to include in the TV programme *It'll Be Alright on the Night*.

In around 1980 or 1981, Diane and I bought our first personal computer for home use, a Commodore 64, which we later upgraded to the Commodore Amiga. I found them strangely fascinating, but confess to only really using them for playing games at that stage, getting hooked on one known as Maxwell's Magic Hammer. I knew they had word processing capabilities but at that time I simply didn't comprehend what an increasingly important role they would play throughout the remainder of my working and personal life. It was in Winchester that a desktop computer first appeared in my office and, with very minimal in-house training, my first attempts at using it were fraught with problems. Not appreciating the difference between 'save' and 'save as', I would create a word document, hit the 'save' button and then immediately lose it. Where had it been saved to? I gradually got used to using a computer and now have a real interest in them, marvelling at their capabilities. Lecturing is now so much easier with PowerPoint than it was when I had to prepare and use transparencies and overhead acetates.

It was also while in Carmarthen and subsequently throughout my career to the present that I developed my interest in goat health and welfare, eventually becoming an Honorary Vet to the British Goat Society.

My youngest daughter Jessica was born in Glangwili General Hospital, Carmarthen, on 25 May 1984. Sadly, my marriage to Diane floundered and we eventually separated and divorced. In 1994, I married Gerry, whose two daughters Nicola and Kimberley were originally at the same Peniel School as Maddy and Jessica before Diane subsequently moved away with them to Gloucestershire. In the same year, Gerry and I moved to the village of Colden Common, near Winchester, where we still live today.

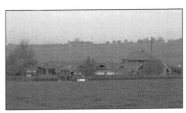

View of the Winchester Regional Laboratory in the Hampshire countryside.

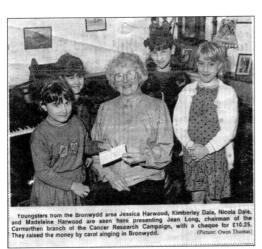

Youngsters from the Bronwydd area Jessica Harwood, Kimberley Dale, Nicola Dale, and Madeleine Harwood are seen here presenting Jean Long, chairman of the Carmarthen branch of the Cancer Research Campaign, with a cheque for £10.25. They raised the money by carol singing in Bronwydd.   (Picture: Owen Thomas)

My daughters and stepdaughters after their successful carol-singing evening.

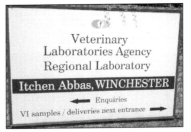

AHVLA Regional Laboratory Winchester entrance sign.

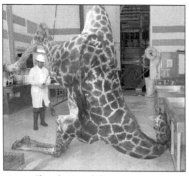

A giraffe submitted for post-mortem examination – not an easy task due to its sheer size!

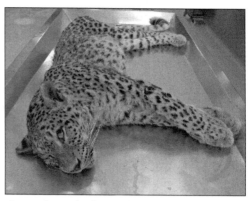

A snow leopard submitted for post-mortem examination from a local zoological park.

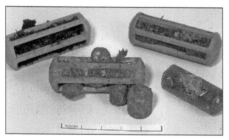

Rumen magnets covered in metallic debris such as tyre wire picked up from the food passing through the stomach.

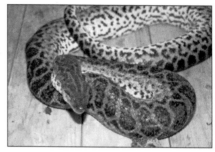

Exotic species such as this present challenges for the pathologist!

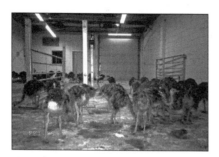

Ostriches at a quarantine centre in Swansea in the 1990s.

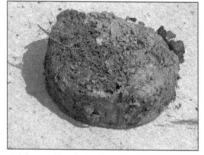

Old tin of high lead content paint exposed when a tree blew over – it caused the death of heifers on a local farm.

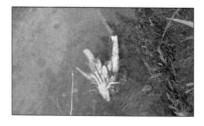

Water dropwort tubers ('Dead Men's Fingers') floating in water following local ditching activity – highly toxic to cattle.

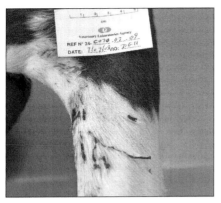

Blood sweating disease in a calf – note the rivulets of blood on the white hair of its limb.

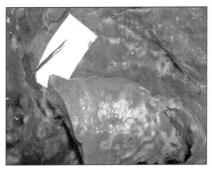

Heart of a cow that died from tyre wire disease – a fragment of wire is embedded in its myocardium.

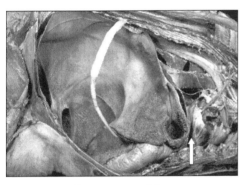

Cross section of a cow prepared for anatomy demonstration – the arrow points to the proximity of the reticulum to the heart.

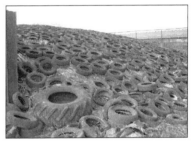

Tyres on a silage clamp that can deteriorate and cause fragments of radial steel to be eaten and penetrate the reticulum.

Chapter 13
Mad Cows and an Englishman

BSE and its ramifications were a major blow for the UK cattle sector. It caused an increasing suspicion of the safety of British beef by the UK consumer and an outright ban on the import of beef, beef products and live cattle from the UK by the remainder of the EU and beyond. The problem was first identified and then categorised, assessed, monitored and eventually controlled during my time at Carmarthen and Winchester, and I was involved from the outset.

I attended a meeting of the BCVA on 7 and 8 July 1987 at the University of Nottingham School of Agriculture. In a session entitled New Diseases, Colin Whitaker, a practitioner from Kent, and Carl Johnson, a VIO from the Wye VI centre, presented a paper entitled *A Neurological Syndrome*. As Carl worked for the same service as me, I had received advance warning of his findings prior to the meeting, but its potential significance then and also at this meeting was not immediately clear. How things changed quite quickly and dramatically!

Colin first called the condition a 'chronic hypersensitivity and incoordination syndrome'. This was based purely on his observations of his first and subsequent cases. It was on 25 April 1985 that Colin was first asked by one of his clients to consider a Holstein Friesian cow that was presented for examination because of a change in its normal character. It had become aggressive and reportedly charged madly around the farm when disturbed. Rectal examination at that time confirmed cystic ovaries and this was thought to be the underlying reason for the unusual behaviour. Hormonal treatment for these cystic ovaries was successful, in that the ovaries returned to normal, but the behaviour continued. Nervous acetonaemia, linked to low circulating blood glucose and a subsequent build-up in the blood of ketones causing unusual nervous signs, was also considered, but again there was no response to treatment. No further treatment was considered appropriate and a tentative diagnosis of a brain tumour or brain abscess was made. The cow was eventually slaughtered on 26 July 1985, exactly three months after it was first examined.

The clinical signs described by Colin are given below and remained remarkably consistent throughout the many cases that were recorded over the next few years. These signs included:

- Progressive hyperaesthesia and incoordination lasting from four weeks to many months.
- A marked change in both character and behaviour.
- Cows become reluctant to enter the milking parlour and when made to enter do so in an exaggerated rush.
- Hypersensitivity to sounds and touch develops.
- Aggression to other cows and to handlers develops.
- Affected cows repeatedly kick in the parlour and become dangerous to milk.
- Cows develop a stiff, slightly stilted, gait on the hind limbs.
- The back is arched slightly and the head often held at an awkward angle with the ears erect.
- There is a fine muscle tremor, particularly over the flanks.
- Some cows will grind their teeth.
- Some cows will lick themselves.
- When cows are rushed on a slippery surface they will often move so fast that they slip and fall, but continue to scrabble along on their knees.
- As the condition progresses cows become recumbent for increasing periods of time, but often show aggressive movements of their head when approached.
- No treatment is effective and cases progress to slaughter on humane grounds.

On the farm where Colin saw his first case, which he considered a one-off, a further, similar case was seen on 9 January 1986. A third cow showing early signs was sent for slaughter by the farmer on 6 February 1986, cow four developed signs while at grass in July 1986 and this was followed by a bull on 19 September 1986.

There had been extensive laboratory testing undertaken and a long list of possible differential diagnoses had been explored but all to no avail and there was still no definitive diagnosis. In the autumn of 1986, as cases were being seen on other farms in the area, cows began to be transported live to the Central Veterinary Laboratory at Weybridge, in Surrey, for more detailed clinical and post-mortem examination.

Eventually, when the brains of cases six, seven and eight were examined in detail histologically, a diagnosis was made. This was a genuinely new disease in cattle presenting as bilaterally symmetric spongiform change to the neuropil part of the brain – literally small holes being evident in the cells of the brain nuclei. Brain homogenates were also prepared and on examination under the electron microscope revealed abnormal fibrils or deposits in brain tissue.

In retrospect, this may seem like a slow process but it is not until a series of cases occur showing the same signs that, as a veterinary surgeon, you begin to wonder if you are experiencing something new. There is a tendency initially to consider each case as a one-off until the number of these begins to increase. It is to Colin's credit that he persevered with this investigation, which began a chain of events that was to continue for the next few years.

It was on 31 October 1987 that the first report appeared in a paper in a peer-reviewed journal, the *Veterinary Record*, with Weybridge pathologist Gerald Wells as the lead author. This focused very much on the pathology of the condition following detailed examination of cases from Kent (previously described by Carl Johnson), but also from other locations, particularly the south-west of England. The pathology was complex and vacuolation (hole formation in brain tissue when viewed down the microscope) was the significant and consistent feature, together with the demonstration of the abnormal fibrils – referred to as scrapie-associated fibrils.

These same authors also began to compare the pathology they were recognising with other known conditions, the so-called spongiform encephalopathies. The most widely recognised of these is the condition referred to as scrapie that affects sheep and goats and which, at that time, was a relatively common problem in the UK sheep sector, having been recognised for around 200 years in the UK. Other conditions with a similar pathological appearance were chronic wasting disease, which affects certain breeds of deer and is reported mainly in the USA, and transmissible mink encephalopathy which affects mink, again principally in the USA.

Of greater concern was the pathological similarity to neurological diseases affecting humans, notably Creutzfeldt-Jakob disease (CJD), a sporadic problem reported in the UK and worldwide, and Kuru, a condition confined to certain cannibalistic tribes in New Guinea.

The UK press had already picked up reports of this condition and first local and subsequently national news bulletins were describing the condition, which had been termed Mad Cow Disease by the media. A short clip of a typical case was archived by the BBC and shown each time the disease was mentioned. The film was of an advanced case on a Devon farm that began with the cow trembling severely and then collapsing and falling sideways as it tried to move away. It was an upsetting piece of film that really fired up the general public and thus began a decline in beef sales as the full picture began to emerge.

There had been intense activity within the state veterinary service. Pathologists at Weybridge had characterised the pathological lesions and identified possible infectious material (the so-called scrapie-associated fibrils). The genetics of the early cases was studied in detail. Could there be an inherited susceptibility? Was there any shared ancestry, specifically as the cases were almost totally confined in the early stages to Holstein Friesian cattle and most breeding was undertaken by artificial insemination? Could these be the offspring of one possibly defective bull? There were no significant findings and although this line of reasoning was pursued for some time, no common ancestry could be identified.

It was to the increasingly important science of epidemiology that the focus then switched. Epidemiology is the study (or the science of the study) of the patterns, causes and effects of health and disease conditions in defined populations. It was in June 1987, that my personal involvement began when I was one of four VIOs drafted into south-west England and based at the Langford laboratory. Our task was to visit those farms where the first 200 cases had been identified and to fill in a long questionnaire for each case/farm, with each taking around two to three hours to complete.

The questionnaire asked some basic questions about the farm structure, including the number of cattle, breed, age structure of the herd and whether it was closed or buying in cattle. Further questions then covered the cases that had occurred to check they fitted the disease profile we had or whether there were any as yet unrecognised features. We then had to collect the breeding data surrounding each case, including the name of the dam or sire and further back if possible. We also had to list the identification (ear tag numbers) of any cattle purchased in the past six months which were to be checked with other farms similarly affected.

Questions then moved to the cow nutrition. We were trying to find out the typical ration being fed, but requesting details of each individual feed constituent including the manufacturer and supplier with relevant batch numbers where available. We recorded any other supplements used, such as mineral licks and blocks or silage additives. We discussed the pasture management, requesting fertiliser and other top dressing products that may have been applied to the herbage, again including batch numbers.

We then turned our attention to pharmaceutical products, looking specifically at the medicine book records of any cases that we were aware of, gathering details of all products used including manufacturer and batch numbers where available. Any farm treatment and prophylaxis (prevention) regimes were explored, including vaccines, hormonal preparations used in fertility management, antibiotics, wormers, flukicides (to manage liver fluke), ectoparasiticides (treating external parasites such as lice or mange), dry cow and lactating cow intramammary preparations used to treat and prevent mastitis, teat dips used to sanitise teats in the parlour and so on. No stone was left unturned in our efforts to identify any common factors that might be partly or wholly responsible for this new and worrying condition.

One of the very early suspicions that came to the surface was the increasingly widespread use of insecticidal, usually organophosphorus (OP), ear tags to prevent biting flies irritating grazing cattle. There were known reports of often tenuous links between exposure to OPs and the display of neurological signs and this had received widespread publicity following occupational exposure to OPs in certain sheep dips. As the tag was a relatively new innovation (as was BSE) and as it was placed very close to the brain tissue in the ear, with the potential opportunity for the chemicals impregnated in the tag to diffuse along peripheral nerves to the brain, it was considered seriously. However, it was obvious there must have been other factors since many thousands of cattle had these tags in their ears and were perfectly healthy.

Genetics factors were also quickly ruled out as extensive studies failed to demonstrate any consistent genetic links between known cases. Although early cases occurred in Holstein Friesian cattle, cases began to occur in other pure breeds, such as Ayrshire and Guernsey cattle and also in cross-breeds such as Hereford X Friesian.

There was also no evidence to suggest the disease had been introduced to the UK from abroad. It had undoubtedly developed within the UK and it seemed most likely after all the analysis had been completed that it came from a single, common source.

There was pathological evidence that the aetiology (cause) of BSE was related to scrapie of sheep, a condition for which there had never been a suggestion it had ever crossed the species barrier to infect cattle under normal farming management procedures. At this time, it was also apparent that around 20 per cent of the cattle farms affected with BSE had no contact with sheep at all, so natural transmission seemed highly unlikely. However, further more specific examination of brain homogenates also gave compelling evidence that the causative agent was one and the same. The next step was to undertake transmission studies. Could scrapie-infected brain material cause BSE signs in cattle to develop after they were experimentally infected? This was immediately problematic in that the incubation period of this group of diseases is long, so any experiment set up might need to run for years and not weeks or months before any findings became apparent.

Attention was now being directed towards the food-borne hypothesis. The incidence was immediately noted to be higher in dairy than in beef cattle and dairy cows are fed more manufactured feed throughout their lives by comparison.

Commercial concentrates, either finished rations such as pelleted calf feed and dairy cow cake or protein supplements used in home mixed rations, were fed at some stage to all the cases for which accurate clinical records were available.

Further investigation into the potential constituents of animal origin was undertaken and both meat and bone meal and also tallow were regularly incorporated after being rendered. Rendering is a process that converts waste animal tissue into stable, value-added material. Such waste may originate from abattoirs and food processing plants but, significantly, would undoubtedly contain material of sheep origin that was being fed to cattle.

At that time there was no clear explanation why around 1982, when it was thought the early adult BSE cases would have been infected, most likely as calves, the opportunity arose for the scrapie agent to survive the rendering process and become incorporated in the finished feed product. It was known, however, that the organism was highly resistant to heat and chemical destruction. There were a number of hypotheses at the time, including a dramatic increase in sheep numbers in the UK over the past few years and a parallel increase in the incidence of scrapie. It also became apparent that more sheep heads, and hence potentially infected brains, were then being rendered than previously, coinciding with a greater inclusion of casualty and condemned sheep material as a result of a reduction in the number of knacker's yards in the UK. Further investigation of the rendering process itself also appeared to suggest the material was being rendered at a lower temperature and/or for a shorter period of time than previously, coinciding with changes in the way the fat was handled and rendered.

The conclusion was reached very early in the course of the outbreak due to some excellent collaborative work across the state veterinary service showing that it was the scrapie agent surviving changes in the rendering process and being inadvertently fed to cattle that initiated this outbreak. SVS and MAFF (as it was then) did receive some unfair criticism from both the media and independent reviews but being on the inside gave me a real understanding of just how these investigations were initiated and handled. There were many individual contributors who took the lead, but the number of VIO and VO hours spent chasing up these first few cases gave them the support that was required to deliver their findings, and I played my part.

We knew the incubation period was long (years) – thus we also knew that even if control measures were put in place to plug the leak of scrapie material into the cattle feed, there could be hundreds if not thousands of cattle potentially incubating the disease, and so it was that the epidemic continued.

It was estimated the first case may have been seen as early as April 1985 but many vets in practice were of the opinion at that time that they had seen cases much earlier than this, and I admit to being one of them. As a former practitioner myself, I could certainly think back to individual cows I had been called to see that were displaying unexplained aggression, or a reluctance to enter the parlour. These were often culled and disposed of, with no laboratory backup, and the evidence would have been lost. There were also theories that we may have always had BSE in cattle in the UK, but running at such a low level as not to raise suspicion. However, I think that over the years this theory has been largely dispelled.

The epidemic began to increase slowly towards the end of the summer of 1987 and by September 1987 we were confirming the cases at the rate of around 60 a month. The highest incidence in these early cases occurred in Kent and Hampshire but sporadic cases were now being seen across the country. Both the veterinary and farming press were regularly now running articles on this new condition and as a result both veterinary practitioners, farmers and stockmen were being urged to look out for the disease, with information on the main clinical presenting signs being widely disseminated.

Before the disease was made notifiable (i.e. there is a legal obligation to report a suspicion of disease to the relevant authority), the VIOs at the VI centres around the country investigated suspect cases reported to them by their local veterinary practices. I had been out on a farm in the Cardigan area investigating a serious outbreak of calf pneumonia with the farm's own vet. As we were about to leave the farm, the owner asked us to look at one of his cows which was behaving strangely.

Knowing the presenting signs of BSE, having seen confirmed cases when working in south-west England, I asked for the cow to be let out of its box and into a yard for us to examine. It was a typical case of BSE, displaying almost all of the signs that were expected. It was twitching violently and its ears were rotating like helicopter blades. It seemed terrified of us, yet it had previously been a quiet cow. What has stuck in my mind to this day, however, was the animal's next action. A length of hosepipe was stretched across the yard and this cow walked up to it, looking increasingly startled as it approached. It walked along to its left and then to its right, apparently working out how to get over a hose that was no more than 2 cm thick. It then proceeded to try to jump over the hosepipe and literally fell over it. This had to be BSE. The cow was sent for slaughter, the head came into the laboratory in Carmarthen and the condition was confirmed. This was the first case of this disease in Wales and eventually featured as the main story on the local news bulletins.

Initially, all the histopathological examination was undertaken by the pathologists at Weybridge but they quickly became overwhelmed as the cases continued to escalate. It was imperative that they worked out a rapid screening test and that others were trained up to help speed diagnoses through the system for the sake of anxious waiting farmers. Following their examination of many brains, it was apparent there were certain parts of the brain that were consistently showing lesions. The most consistent of these was the nucleus of the solitary tract, where the characteristic vacuolation could be clearly seen. I was selected to become one of the primary BSE histopathology readers and spent time at Weybridge becoming familiar with the techniques. I returned to Carmarthen and began reading slides prepared from the brains of suspect cows.

Suspect cows were examined on farm by a VO or VIO and this became a more formal approach after the disease was made notifiable. If confirmed on clinical grounds, the affected cow was destroyed on the farm with barbiturate. We needed the brain intact, so it could not be shot. The carcass was then removed by a local haulier and in the early days taken to either a knacker's yard or a hunt kennel. Later, cows were sent to dedicated incineration sites, a number of which were built solely for this purpose.

The head was removed and delivered to us at the Carmarthen VI centre and to other VI centres around the country. At that time we had to remove the entire brain, which was hard work. The cow's skull is thick and after it was held in a vice the top was taken off by using a hacksaw and crowbar. This exposed the underlying brain, which was then removed and placed in a white pot containing formol saline to prevent any further decay, labelled with the cow/case details and stored ready for processing.

At that time, we wore our normal PM boiler suits and aprons with no other protective face covering and we removed hundreds of brains dressed that way. As the health risks became more apparent, and particularly as health and safety policies became more widely adopted, we had to wear ever increasing personal protective equipment (PPE). As the epidemic continued, I had to wear an airstream helmet and visor which enclosed my head completely, with a separate, battery-operated stream of air blowing over my face. We also wore cut-proof gloves under our normal protective gloves and were even provided with chain mail aprons. In retrospect, I suspect we were all lucky but if ever there was an occupational risk of humans picking up this infection then we must have been at the front of the queue. We were handling infected brain material with very little overall protection!

The technique was also refined so that the part of the brain required for examination (the obex – the hindbrain beneath the cerebellum and attached to the spinal cord) could be removed through a hole through which the spinal cord leaves the skull, known as the foramen magnum. This was a far easier approach with a greatly reduced risk of splashes or aerosols being created with potentially infected brain tissue.

We could cope initially but as the numbers increased – and Carmarthen serves a particularly densely populated cattle area, hence the number of BSE cases rapidly escalated – we dedicated a whole room to BSE. This was a former storage room at the back of the laboratory with no heating. Once each week I spent time opening each of the white pots in which brains that had been removed had been sitting during a period of fixation. This work was carried out in a safety cabinet due to the large amount of formalin fumes created. I had to slice up the brain tissue and specifically select a portion of the obex, including the *calamus scriptorius,* of around 3 mm in thickness and place it in a histology processing cassette. The process of preparing a microscope slide to enable the examination to take place was all undertaken in another part of the laboratory by a member of the technical staff and I did not see the material again until this slide was brought to my room. During the processing, my selected tissue was embedded in wax and then, using a piece of equipment referred to as a microtome (literally a modified and very refined bacon slicer), a section of brain tissue only one to two cells thick was prepared and placed onto the microscope slide. This tissue was then fixed and stained with two dyes known as haematoxylin and eosin (so called H&E), so that the nuclei of the cells stained a bluish colour and the cell cytoplasm a pink colour.

I began by reading only a small number each week, but at the height I was processing up to 200 slides each week. The number of negative cases was very low as the signs were so typical that very few non-BSE cases were slaughtered inadvertently.

BBC Wales became intensely interested in what we were doing in relation to BSE as farming is an extremely important part of the Welsh economy. Its film crews visited us on a number of occasions and archive footage of me in my cold 'brain room' cutting the sections and sitting at my microscope looking at stained sections of BSE brains regularly accompanied any item in which the condition was referred to. BBC Wales also interviewed me twice sitting in my office. This would not happen today as media enquiries are dealt with by the Defra press office but at that time we were given a fairly free rein in how we approached such requests. It was also my first encounter with investigative journalism and my first interview was heavily edited and rearranged, so that my answer to one question was deliberately attributed to another so as to make a final, emphatic point. I had been asked what I thought the most useful next step could be and after some thought I had stated a test to use in the live cow would be most useful. This phrase was actually part of another answer I had given.

By the time the epidemic began to die down it had become a huge news story, not only in the UK, but around the world as other countries recognised they also had the disease. Some of these cases undoubtedly occurred in cattle we had exported before the worldwide ban came into place but others were due to similar practices in these countries. The UK outbreak statistics tell us we have had a total of 183,841 confirmed cases, far more than any other country such as France (900), Republic of Ireland (1,353) and Portugal (875). Even Japan (26), and Canada (17) reported cases.

It took a long time to get on top of this epidemic, which was controlled mainly by a ban on the inclusion of any protein or protein derivative of animal origin being fed to ruminants. The ban was largely successful but, due to the long incubation period, inevitably took a long time to show the results that government and the population at large wished to see. However, cases did decline and by 2014 BSE had virtually been eradicated. No matter what criticism has been levelled at MAFF /Defra over its handling of this crisis, I do take pride in what we achieved. Many of us put a considerable amount of time and effort into getting on top of this disease and the constant criticism used to get me down and I suspect it was not always easy for those making the important decisions at the top to deal with.

Running alongside the epidemic in cattle was a similar outbreak affecting cats and referred to as FSE (feline spongiform encephalopathy). We at Carmarthen and also in Winchester received domestic cats for examination along similar lines to cattle. These were almost certainly infected via scrapie contamination of cat food. We also saw a number of incidents at zoos and when in Winchester I removed the brains from a lion and a tiger from a local collection, which also saw a number of cases in its antelopes.

It was, of course, the human tragedy of variant CJD that brought home the overall seriousness of the condition and the farming practices that had preceded it. We had more than 170 cases confirmed in the UK, many of these in young people. These also now appear to have been curtailed.

On my way to Defra headquarters I regularly walked past a constant reminder of my involvement in the BSE epidemic. On the embankment opposite the Palace of Westminster on the wall outside St Thomas's hospital is a plaque which reads:

'In loving memory of the victims of human BSE (vCJD), always in our thoughts. (Human BSE Foundation)'.

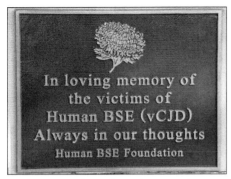

A plaque outside St Thomas's Hospital, opposite the Houses of Parliament in London.

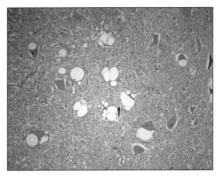

The histopathological appearance of the brain confirming BSE – note the small "holes" in brain tissue (spongiform change).

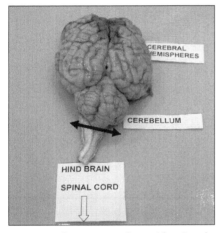

Anatomy of a ruminant brain (sheep) – the black line indicates the plane in which sections were taken for BSE tests.

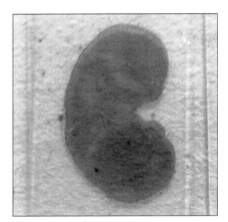

An 'H & E' stained section of the obex ready for histological examination.

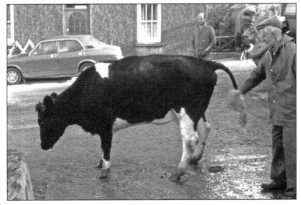

This cow was the first case of BSE confirmed in Wales taken while I was working in Carmarthen.

Chapter 14

A National Crisis Unfolds – I Head Out onto the Front Line

The year 2001 was memorable worldwide for the devastating and deadly attacks on the World Trade Center in New York on 11 September.

It was also the year that foot-and-mouth disease arrived in the UK, creating its own unfolding catalogue of despair for the UK farming industry, the countryside, the tourist industry and the UK economy and costing in excess of £8 billion. FMD is a highly infectious disease affecting predominantly cloven hoofed animals, such as cattle, sheep, goats, pigs and deer. The disease itself could be described in many cases as mild, with only a fever and minimal lesions. That said it can also cause very dramatic and intensely painful lesions, including a complete loss of the epithelial covering of the tongue or the shelling of the hoof. Both of these leave raw and painful underlying tissue exposed. The classic signs are, as the name suggests, confined to the mouth, in which vesicles (or blisters) develop on the tongue, gums and lips. These can quickly burst leaving raw lesions, which in turn lead to the salivation that is often the first indication that an animal has the disease. Similar lesions develop on the soft tissue around the claws, leading to varying degrees of lameness depending on the severity and number of digits affected.

I was 17 when the last really severe outbreak of FMD occurred. The first case was identified in Shropshire in October 1967, and was followed by an epidemic which resulted in the slaughter of 442,000 animals. Most of these were slaughtered to prevent further spread of the disease. This method of control has received much criticism, but has nevertheless continued into the more recent outbreaks. It is important to point out, however, that in the absence of a vaccination programme, it was the only practical method of halting the spread of this highly infectious disease. We had no cases in Church Lench where I grew up, but Shropshire was close by, and we farms with susceptible livestock did receive regular visits by the

Ministry of Agriculture vets, all wearing the long black macs and black sou'westers that seemed to represent the doom that accompanied each visit.

During my time in practice in Blandford Forum, there was a brief incursion of FMD into the UK in March 1981 but it was confined to the Isle of Wight, having spread from a small outbreak in northern France. Its ability to spread via wind and air movements, as indicated by its crossing from mainland Europe, put the UK mainland at risk and as we were a practice near the south coast, we were on high alert. Disinfectant-soaked straw mats were laid down at the entrance to the practice and at the entrance to many farms and our visits quickly began to dry up as farms shut themselves down hoping FMD would not spread. We were aware of our responsibility to set an example to our clients and our cars were cleaned once or twice each day, including the wheels and wheel arches. We simply could not be seen to disregard the risks. Luckily, this incursion never spread to the mainland.

As I have already outlined, my first personal experience of the disease occurred early in my career as a veterinary investigation officer when as part of my training I spent time at the Institute of Animal Health at Pirbright in Surrey, where the World Reference Foot-and-Mouth Disease Laboratory is based. On this same site, research work is also undertaken on a number of other exotic diseases that we do not see in the UK, but remain on the lookout for. These included swine fever, African swine fever, rinderpest, and sheep and goat pox. With FMD, these make up part of the list of notifiable diseases in the UK and EU. Essentially, any livestock keeper or veterinary surgeon who suspects any of these diseases to be present in live animals must by law report it to the relevant government department (previously MAFF but now Defra), which must investigate as a matter of urgency. Such an obligation also rests with other authorities, such as market inspectors and those inspecting livestock prior to slaughter and after slaughter in abattoirs. It was in an abattoir that the 2001 outbreak was first identified.

My training experience at Pirbright did have a profound effect on me, firstly by making sure that I never forgot the importance of considering these diseases in any sick live animal I examined or dead animal on which I undertook a post-mortem examination. It was a subliminal assessment, one in time I didn't even have to think about. The strict biosecurity surrounding Pirbright and the great emphasis on the potential for these diseases to spread rapidly through our livestock was also a wake-up call as to what would happen if such a disease was overlooked. Sadly, it was this very feature of FMD that led to the 2001 epidemic and the race to catch up with a disease that had had a major head start.

One of my biggest frustrations during 2001, when I was often working right at the heart of the outbreak, was the constant media attention. This was often presented in such a manner as to resemble a witch-hunt against those of us charged with controlling the problem. This was not necessarily aimed at my level but nevertheless constant criticism and undermining control measures put in place can be very demoralising for all concerned. Equally, those not involved formed their opinions mainly from the media coverage, so even my close friends and family were critical of how things were being conducted. In reality, we were working long exhausting hours doing our best to implement control policies and I became increasingly fed up with spending almost all my time away from the epidemic defending what I was doing while I was working in the heart of it.

It all began on Monday, 19 February 2001 in an abattoir in Brentwood, Essex, when a member of staff expressed concern about a group of sows that had been held in the lairage over the weekend. This concern was immediately passed on to Craig Kirby, the resident veterinary surgeon. He could not rule out a vesicular disease (either swine vesicular disease or foot-and-mouth) based on the clinical signs and immediately telephoned the local State Veterinary Service. It sent out two veterinary officers, one of whom had experience of FMD in Greece. They could not rule out either of these diseases and took samples that were immediately taken to Pirbright. FMD was confirmed and the State Veterinary Service and the experts at Pirbright immediately began to assess the situation, initially identifying and investigating the farm of origin of the pigs and then the extent of the spread. It quickly became apparent that the disease, although identified in Essex, did not originate from that locality. The lesions in the sows were already a few days old and must have developed either in transit or when on their farm of origin, which was many miles away in Northumberland.

At the time, I was junior vice-president of the BCVA and was due to take over the presidency in April 2001 but all this was to change dramatically. The chief veterinary officer (CVO), Jim Scudamore, and his headquarters staff convened what was referred to as a stakeholder meeting at MAFF. This was an approach that was becoming more widespread, when effectively those with knowledge of the industry or those whose livelihood depended on it were asked to attend or send representatives for a briefing and update; it was also to gauge views to assist in the development of policy. Within days of the disease being confirmed, there was already much activity within MAFF and the first such meeting took place.

I represented the BCVA and joined around 25 to 30 stakeholders including people from farming unions, local authorities, veterinary associations, the police and welfare charities. I clearly remember the very sombre mood in the room as the outbreak data began to appear and was relayed to us. I also recall pieces of paper being passed to the CVO, each one of which signalled yet another new incident that had been identified as the meeting was taking place.

None of us realised that, far from being a simple outbreak, the disease had already got well ahead of us. It had spread from the original index case to more than 50 premises, from Devon in the south to Dumfries and Galloway in the north, and the chase had to begin in earnest to overtake and control the spread of this most infectious of diseases. It was spread so rapidly by the unprecedented and uncontrolled number of sheep movements around the UK at that time.

Working as I did for MAFF, it was inevitable I would be called on very quickly to begin tackling and controlling the outbreak. Somewhat ironically, I had already agreed to spend the weekend after the outbreak was confirmed on BCVA 'duty' in London with Gerry, but luckily I didn't get the call until the Monday after I returned home. This weekend consisted of a two-night stay at Claridge's Hotel, a reception at the House of Lords, dinner at the Four Seasons Hotel in Park Lane, a corporate day at the England-Scotland rugby international at Twickenham and dinner at Claridge's. It was certainly tough at times being on the BCVA presidential ladder. However, discussions between vets throughout this weekend were inevitably taken up by FMD.

We never had any disease confirmed in Hampshire throughout the epidemic so, as a result, I spent almost my entire time living and working away from home, spending weeks in local hotels close to my FMD work base.

I was first asked to work out of the Leicester Animal Health Office as there had been a series of outbreaks in the Nuneaton area that needed to be investigated and controlled. I travelled up to Leicester to be there for the 8.30am situation report and update. I had brought my own protective clothing with me but was also kitted out with all the equipment I needed. These included disposable overalls, which had replaced the black macs and sou'westers so firmly engrained in my mind from my childhood memories of fowl pest. We also had disposable gloves, sampling equipment to enable laboratory testing, pads of dedicated FMD forms (and carbon paper for duplicating copies), gallons of disinfectant and all the necessary OS maps that we might need to cover our area, which was totally unfamiliar to me. We had no satnav at that time and map-reading became an essential skill for us all to develop if we were to find some very isolated and remote farms over the coming days, weeks and months.

The overall control of the national response to such an outbreak comes from the headquarters, where a dedicated team is set up to staff the NDECC (National Disease Emergency Control Centre) and in which I was based during the 2007 outbreak. There is also a locally-based field operations centre set up usually at an animal health office – such as Leicester. This in turn is referred to as the LDECC (Local Disease Emergency Control Centre). Within each LDECC, a number of teams are established made up of representatives from existing state veterinary service staff (who take on the lead roles), veterinary practitioners who are drafted in to help, field and office staff from other government departments drafted in on secondment, RSPCA, police, auctioneers (who value stock prior to slaughter), slaughtermen and local authority staff. The teams also included the army, which was called in as the magnitude of the problem became apparent.

The team I was to join was referred to as the surveillance team and was investigating suspected new on-farm cases (or report cases) and visiting farms within the 'at-risk area' to check for new disease. Once disease had been confirmed on a farm there would be another team going on to the farm to arrange valuation and slaughter/disposal of infected stock, with yet another team following behind them to clean and disinfect the now empty premises to remove any residual infection. Another group, referred to as the epidemiology team, drew up lists of farms that fell in designated at-risk areas (usually those within a 3 or 5 km radius of an infected farm) that were each put under restriction by issuing a Form C licence. There was already a national ban on farm animal movements, but the Form C restriction effectively declared a zone with temporary, but even more restrictive, control measures as a result of infection confirmed nearby.

One of these Form C restrictions was to be visited every 48 hours by a veterinary inspector of MAFF and this was the category I was initially placed in with volunteer veterinary surgeons from both the UK and, increasingly as the epidemic proceeded, from overseas. So it was that on my first day in that role I was given a list of livestock units to visit. It is important to emphasise these restrictions applied to all holdings with susceptible livestock, including hobby keepers, zoos and even theme parks with a pet corner that might have only two goats. They all had to be visited. Our task on each visit was to discuss and assess the effectiveness of control measures put in place to keep infection out and advise on any apparent inadequacies. We then had to inspect all the susceptible livestock on each farm to ensure they were fit and healthy and specifically showed no signs of FMD. We had to be scrupulous about not spreading and thus introducing infection ourselves, so our cars were always parked well outside the farm gate. All of these had a long disinfected straw mat at the entrance which was designed to disinfect the full circumference of any wheel passing over it. We often donned our full protective gear on the roadside, before gathering together whatever equipment we might need and setting off up the drive to the farm.

My approach was consistently to look at all the susceptible stock, initially by observation while they were undisturbed and more likely to show signs of ill health. I then went into each pen, building or field to walk among the group, requesting a closer examination of any individual that showed any signs that caused me concern. This was always much easier with housed animals but was often a nightmare when one wished to examine a lame sheep in a large field. If I was satisfied all livestock looked fit and healthy, I would remind the owner that my visit was only able to confirm that all was OK on the day of my visit. As FMD is incredibly infectious, and as the incubation period is short, it is imperative they remained vigilant between me leaving and their next visit. I also reminded the owner what to look out for and how to get in touch with us.

As my car was parked away from the farm and any water supply, I invariably had to carry a bucket of water back to my car to make up my disinfectant. It was then a case of carrying out a full clean up. Disposable overalls were removed (and I wore these over my waterproof gear to keep them clean) and plunged in disinfectant before being placed in a bag for later disposal. I then disinfected my boots, placed all other items such as gloves into my disposal bag and got ready to move off to my next farm. When all my calls were complete and I was content that I had seen only healthy animals, I phoned back to the LDECC to check there were no outstanding tasks to complete in my area. I then returned to Leicester to complete my paperwork.

Unsurprisingly, many livestock keepers were apprehensive about these routine visits by vets. Many felt that they were not being trusted to report disease themselves, and others were just plain scared that we would bring disease onto their farms ourselves. Most accepted that it was inevitable that we had to gain entry to their farms, but others were far more vociferous in their opposition, with some even threatening violence if we set foot inside their gates.

Although I didn't know it, I had been given two of these 'problem farms' in my first two days, but had no problem gaining entry to either and undertaking the tasks that I needed to perform. I was then asked if I would visit one particularly awkward dairy farmer, who so far had not allowed anyone onto his premises. We met at the gate, and he made it very clear to me that he was not going to allow me to set foot on his farm that day. We discussed the implications of this – that I would have to get a policeman to accompany me, which would present an added risk. He had driven down to the farm gate on his tractor, so I suggested that he could drive me around the farm so that I could at least see his cattle – and I would not be setting foot on the farm, as he requested. As a result, we developed, over that and subsequent visits, a regime which he was satisfied with (he had, in part, got his own way) but which also allowed me to do my job. I literally never set foot on his farm, spending my time on the towbar of the tractor, while he backed me to the edges of the yards and slowly walked each cow past me. Any that I was concerned about were then brought up to the tractor for me to examine. I would step off the tractor onto a wooden pallet at the front of the cattle crush to examine the cow, before stepping back onto the tractor again.

The LDECC were somewhat surprised by my approach, but genuinely agreed that the task in hand was being undertaken satisfactorily; if anything, having the cows walked past me slowly may even have meant I did a better job than when I walked in amongst them on other farms. I think the fact that I was a mature, large animal vet able to prove my competence must have helped – farmers can be a suspicious lot, and can be particularly suspicious of vets they do not know coming onto their farms and making decisions about their livestock and, by definition, about their livelihood.

This task was far from easy on some premises. As an example, one was a large pig unit with around 3,000 housed animals in which the disease was often difficult to recognise. Luckily there was also a beef fattening unit on this farm, with shared staff and equipment. In this outbreak, cattle appeared to show more pronounced signs, so my first stop was always the cattle yards. If the cows were all fit and healthy, I had some indication that the pigs would also be OK. Inspecting 3,000 pigs took time as I had to be confident that I had at least 'seen' every animal before I left. We had to catch and examine every one that was either lame or showed any lesions on the muzzle or was salivating (which pigs often do). I had a marker spray to ensure I could recognise these again at my next visit to assess progress.

On my third day, I visited a smallholding in a series of fairly run-down buildings at the roadside that housed around 20 to 30 beef fatteners. It was not a well-run farm and many of the cattle seen were not in very good condition. I ran a few of them through a crush and found three with mouth lesions and two more that were lame. The lesions all looked chronic and fairly longstanding with mainly ulceration of the tongue and gums and what looked like 'foul in the foot', a recognised foot problem. I was 99 per cent certain that in the absence of the current FMD concerns, I would suspect mucosal disease (causing ulceration in the mouth) and foul, but could I be 100 per cent certain now? At that time, those of us in the field were able to be suspicious without taking the immediate and very draconian measures that would be brought in as the outbreak continued. I discussed my findings with the NDECC team, suggesting I place the farm under restriction with FMD signs clearly displayed at the gate stating 'no entry', and they agreed. I arranged to return the following morning as by this time it was already getting dark.

I then had the problem of what to do with the owner and his wife as they only had their work clothes with them. I had protective clothing over my clothes that I could easily clean and disinfect. The 'day clothes' of the owner and his wife, however, were both fairly heavily contaminated with faeces and I could not allow them to take these off the farm after I had placed it under restriction. Luckily, their car was parked across the road from the farm, off the premises, therefore it did not require full disinfection. I suggested that I gave them each a paper overall to wear home – leaving their farm clothes on the farm until the next day, when I would either rule out or confirm disease. I then helped them clean and disinfect their boots, disinfected the outside of their car and the foot wells where their dirty boots had been and then sent them off on their way looking like suspects in a serious crime. I returned at first light to re-examine the cattle I had seen the previous day. They were unchanged and there were no further cases evident, so I lifted restrictions immediately.

Sheep presented us with many problems during the 2001 outbreak, mainly due to the very vague signs they often presented. Recognising this as the outbreak progressed, some of my veterinary colleagues working in Cumbria coined a term referred to as 'OMAGOD' (sounding like 'Oh My God', but in reality, the acronym means 'Ovine Mouth and Gum Obscure Disease' – because you open the mouth and suspect you have a case of FMD). There are a number of causes, other than FMD, for sheep getting such lesions – particularly if they are on rough moorland grazing – and as a result, they may mistakenly be taken as suspect FMD. There are also many causes of lameness, most of which I was wholly familiar with.

I visited one smallholding in the Nuneaton area a number of times, and noticed lame sheep at my first visit, all of which I examined. I was quite satisfied that this was a footrot problem, and felt I could rule out FMD, partly due to my alternative diagnosis, but also supported by the absence of any mouth lesions. I finished my FMD 2001 year working at the World Reference Foot and Mouth Disease laboratory at Pirbright, where I had the chance to check up on some of my early cases – and found this farm. It had been slaughtered out with suspect FMD only ten days after I left the area, with a history stating: 'number of lame sheep with typical FMD pathology'. However, all laboratory testing on samples taken was negative – this farm never had FMD! I had the benefit of being familiar with footrot in sheep, and also having seen these particular sheep on more than one occasion. The vet that reported a suspicion of FMD was on the farm for the first time when presented with these same sheep, and may not have had the confidence to diagnose footrot; such were the pressures that were placed on each and every one of us (as I found out myself later in the outbreak). I became aware of a number of other such incidents as the outbreak continued – and accept that it is easy to criticise with hindsight, but it was perhaps inevitable that this would happen as the outbreak rapidly overtook the capabilities of the entire UK veterinary profession, resulting in a need for overseas help.

I arrived back at the hotel each evening feeling both physically and mentally exhausted. From the looks on the faces of the hotel staff, I reeked fairly strongly of disinfectant. To separate the rigours of the day from the evening, I quickly developed a routine, and this began with a soak in the bath to remove the smell of disinfectant, which even after a bath often lingered in your nostrils. I would then phone Gerry to have a chat about our respective days, before heading downstairs for something to eat and drink. As many of the hotel guests were also vets and other professionals working on FMD, there was little else discussed apart from our respective experiences. On reflection, this made it increasingly difficult to relax and this was compounded by a lack of sleep as I never sleep well when away from home.

I am usually a fairly practical, down-to-earth vet, but I hadn't realised how emotionally I was becoming involved until I burst into tears on the phone to Gerry one day (Mothering Sunday in fact) when I realised that life was going on outside my bubble of daily foot-and-mouth and its problems.

The day before, a husband and wife who were joint owners of a smallholding and shop and who were under Form C restrictions had both begun to cry in front of me. I'd had to comfort the owner's wife, who was sobbing on my shoulder. I had just inspected their livestock and everything was clear but they began talking about the impact the restrictions had on them. Their shop was closed, they could not sell any livestock and they had just received two final demands for payment in the post that morning, one of which was for their daughter's hall of residence fees at university. They did not know which way to turn or what to do next and everything was stacked up against them. I believe that many of us working during this dreadful time suffered some form of mental anguish – I know I did – and luckily Gerry recognised this and I came home for a couple of days' break. All staff were given regular breaks and the Working Time Directive was adhered to whenever possible, but those of us working in the field were committed to playing our part in controlling this disease, and many of us knowingly worked much longer stretches without a break than we should have. We had been taught how to deal with the animal-related issues, but I was not a trained counsellor, and this was a role I was trying to perform. Absorbing everyone's problems and trying to offer comfort was taking its toll. I still sometimes well up when I am asked about my experiences, or when I recount a particularly poignant story.

I formed some very strong friendships with other vets at that time. Many of us were living away from home in hotels and spent a lot of time in the hotel bar and restaurant in the evenings. I eventually spent three weeks in the same hotel in Leicester before my next assignment was given out.

As the problem was coming under control in the Leicester/Nuneaton area, it was escalating in other parts of the country, particularly Cumbria and Devon. I was sent to Devon and subsequently went straight from Leicester to Exeter to join the Exeter LDECC, with yet another hotel room waiting for me.

My role in Devon was initially the same as my role in Leicester in that I went out each day undertaking surveillance visits to those farms mainly around Dartmoor that were also under Form C restriction. The LDECC set-up in Exeter was much larger than in Leicester and temporary offices had been erected with a new overflow car park. The epidemic was escalating and as a result there were many more vets, with an increasing number from overseas, volunteering to help. The army had also been drafted in wearing their uniform, which gave them a very visible presence. Over the coming weeks as the crisis deepened, around 2,000 military personnel were eventually deployed at both NDECC and LDECC level mainly in Devon and Cumbria. Their skill in dealing with logistical problems was invaluable and their presence released vets and other animal health personnel to carry out tasks to which they were better suited.

In Leicester, it had been a short drive to the relatively small focus of infection I had been dealing with. Devon, however, is a large county with a heavy livestock presence and, as a result, the distances travelled between the LDECC and my list of farm visits were often long. That was despite the farms themselves being often close together and centred on one village. Devon is a beautiful county. I knew it well having lived and worked in mid-Devon for three years. By the time I arrived, it was early spring and the catkins, daffodils and primroses were all in full show. The early season holidaymakers would have been packing the roads but the county away from the main roads was eerily quiet. Every farm gate was shut, there were no tractors out on the roads and footpaths were closed. As MAFF employees we were very visible, often passing each other as we prepared to enter a farm or disinfected ourselves at the roadside between visits.

The peak of the epidemic occurred during my time in Devon, with the national number of cases escalating to around 50 a day before beginning a gradual decline. It continued well into the autumn, almost six months later, and none of us expected that.

As I drove over the edge of Dartmoor one day, it was hard not to notice the plumes of smoke across the valley on the opposite hillside; I stopped the car and counted six separate plumes. Each of these signified a farm where FMD had been confirmed or which had been slaughtered out as an 'at-risk farm', and the smoke was coming up from the funeral pyre disposing of the animal remains, often burning for days. It is not hard to imagine just how big these funeral pyres could be if you consider that on occasion it could contain hundreds of cattle or on some farms literally thousands of sheep. This process had changed very little from the last FMD outbreak in 1967, and in many ways did seem very out of place in an increasingly modern world.

One of the sections in the FMD manual was completely devoted to the practicalities of constructing and maintaining the funeral pyre, using straw bales and railway sleepers and even napalm. Other methods of disposal are now available should there ever be a need. One of the problems encountered in 2001 was that the number of animals slaughtered rapidly overwhelmed the ability to dispose of them, such that at its peak, there were some 229,775 carcasses awaiting disposal. With the army and its logistics staff, the disposal capacity was doubled and then redoubled with little overall impact (as the numbers slaughtered still exceeded the numbers disposed of) initially, taking nearly six weeks before disposal routes were able to cope with demand. This was achieved mainly by the development and exploitation of mass burial sites, which could then utilise massive industrial machinery, alongside constant lorry movement to and from farms, with disposal in large pits. The largest of these was in Cumbria at Great Orton, but a number of others were set up, including one at Throckmorton in Worcestershire, at an old airfield I could so easily see from my bedroom window as I grew up in Church Lench – it is interesting how coincidences happen!! On-farm burial was considered as an alternative, but due to the potential persistence of the BSE agent in the environment (and BSE was still a problem at that time), it was considered inadvisable to bury cattle over five years of age. As a result of the mass burial sites, and also of the increasingly available commercial incinerator or rendering sites to which adult cattle could be taken, burning on farm by means of these funeral pyres actually ceased in early May 2001.

It is only when with hindsight you look at the statistics of an outbreak that you realise why we had such a problem. Although the UK cattle population between 1967 and 2001 had remained fairly static at 11 to 12 million, the sheep population had increased from around 28 million to more than 40 million in the same period. At the same time, the number of holdings had decreased and the numbers of both sheep and cattle on each livestock unit had also increased, in some cases quite dramatically – therefore each confirmed farm case presented a greater number of animals to examine, slaughter and dispose of. The average number of animals slaughtered on each infected premises during 1967 was 184, compared with 631 in 2001, an increase of more than 40 per cent.

There had been a considerable amount of media interest in how the outbreak was being handled and as the crisis deepened the Prime Minister, Tony Blair, took overall control. One of his visits was to the Exeter LDECC, although none of us working in the field got the opportunity to meet him – we were all out on farms.

For myself, the long days continued with me driving down to my 'patch' going from farm to farm looking for evidence of disease, and perhaps of significance considering the number of farms I visited and the livestock I inspected, I never found a single case that I felt the need to report. I hope this was in part down to my skills and experience as a farm animal vet, in that I was able to diagnose a number of other conditions that mimic FMD. It was well known that at the height of the epidemic, there were many farms slaughtered out as being suspected disease, only for disease to be ruled out on laboratory examination.

We were all staying together in hotels, so inevitably most (if not all) of the discussion over dinner and in the bar was about the problem we were dealing with. It did surprise me that so many newly recruited vets 'found' disease within the first few days of arrival, often on more than one farm – carrying out the same inspection visits that I was. Other experienced colleagues working with me felt much the same; they simply could not all be true cases, yet in the heat of the moment, very few were actually turned down when reported, and were slaughtered out. There were always repercussions, however, as slaughtering out one farm often meant that neighbouring farms (so called contiguous premises) or other farms referred to as 'dangerous contacts', might also then be slaughtered out. The implications could be massive. All cases were discussed with veterinary colleagues in the disease reporting team in Page Street in London, who did their best to prevent 'misdiagnosis' – but it took a brave vet sitting in London to turn down a 'suspect FMD case' reported by an enthusiastic vet standing alongside the animal(s) on the farm.

Sheep again presented me with problems in Devon, as most were out on the hills. I became very fit, walking miles each day to inspect my designated flock. We did regularly use one particular mode of transport that I remember all too well – the quad bike, a four-wheel all-terrain vehicle used widely in rural locations off-road. I was transported round many farms as a passenger sitting on one of the mudguards whilst looking at a sign (clearly displayed in front of me) which stated: 'this machine should not be used for carrying passengers'! I accept that this was a dangerous move on my part, but it was a personal decision made at the time and under pressure to examine a large number of sheep scattered around hundreds of acres. Accidents on farms are all too common, and health and safety for those working on or visiting farms must be a priority.

I had taken Easter weekend off as a break and this in itself presented me with a problem. Here I was driving around Devon surrounded by FMD infected farms and I was now intending to drive back home to Hampshire where there was no disease. I knew I must not under any circumstances bring it back with me. So just before I returned home I visited a carwash in Exeter to give my vehicle a thorough wash down. I then disinfected my wheels and wheel arches with my disinfectant spray that I carried at all times and set off for home. Once I had left the infected area, in the middle of Salisbury Plain, I stopped again in a layby and repeated the disinfectant regime. My car then stayed in the drive at home. I remember both Gerry and my friends commenting on how tired I looked and how much weight I had apparently lost.

The time quickly passed and, as I had been asked to be back on Easter Monday for an 8am brief, I left home around 5.30am, completely unaware this was to become my most memorable day of the outbreak. It began routinely with another list of farms to visit, much the same as my other days in Devon. I completed my round, phoned in, was given the all-clear to return and got back to the LDECC at around 6pm to complete my paperwork. Around 7pm I was asked if I would travel back to Dartmoor to give some support and a second opinion to a young New Zealand female vet who was still on a large farm and unable to decide if she had a problem or not. I eventually arrived on the farm at around 8.30pm, only to be told that there were around 3,000 sheep and 400 cattle at this 'large livestock unit'. The vet was most concerned about some lambs and had already been on the farm for much of the day. As cattle were the best indicators of disease, I decided to examine them first. A number were lame and we ran these through the crush. Most were affected with a condition referred to as digital dermatitis but I was concerned about a few that were lame with no real lesions other than pain around the coronary band where FMD lesions commonly develop.

The sheep flock was in the middle of lambing, so many of the adult ewes were housed and available for me to examine. I found nothing of concern in the adults and then turned my attention to the lambs. Many of these were salivating profusely and had well-developed, mainly fleshy, lesions in their mouth. These were typical in my view of a condition known colloquially as orf, or contagious pustular dermatitis, caused by a pox virus. I was 99 per cent sure this farm did not have FMD but was aware that I could have cattle with digital dermatitis and lambs with orf potentially masking a developing FMD.

At around 11.30pm I phoned the NDECC emergency contact to make my report. I did this along the lines described, and was effectively told that unless I could give a 100% guarantee that I could rule out FMD, the farm would be slaughtered out. This was apparently a 'new policy', implemented in an attempt to get ahead of the outbreak and to cut the risk of missing disease. To be told that I had to be 100% sure was a risk I wasn't prepared to take. I argued that as it was now 11.30pm, nothing would happen anyway until the following morning – so why did we have to make a decision right then? I asked to be allowed to return at first light the next day, or even to stay at the farm overnight and reassess the situation in the morning when the condition would undoubtedly be in a more advanced state, arguing that we would have lost little time overall.

'No', was the answer I was given. Unless I could walk away with a 100 per cent negative report, the farm would be designated as SOS, or slaughter on suspicion. I discussed this with the owners, who agreed reluctantly to this approach, and around midnight I signed the death warrant for all livestock on this farm.

I later found out all lab tests were negative and my diagnoses had been correct. If I'd had the confidence to walk away from the farm and state there was no disease, those animals would have survived and the family would have been spared the anguish of having to watch them being slaughtered the following day. With disease all around them, it was perhaps inevitable they would either have become infected or culled for some other reason, but I will never know and this decision has ranked above all others I have ever made as a vet. I still feel I failed those animals, the young New Zealand vet and the farming family and their dependents.

Having left the farm around 12.30am, I arrived at my hotel at close to 2am (they were used to the odd hours I kept as most of the hotels in the area were full of people working on FMD). It was my longest working day during this crisis, I had been up for 21½ hours and, yes, I was back in the office to complete my paperwork and begin another round at 8.30am.

Shortly after this, and as it was obvious the outbreak was going to continue for a long time, many of the full-time MAFF staff such as myself were moved away from the field visits (there were plenty of what were referred to as the veterinary reserve personnel on the ground). I was asked to join the field epidemiology team on the LDECC and become office-bound helping to track infection, work out the likely course it might take and the associated risk factors. This job lasted precisely one day.

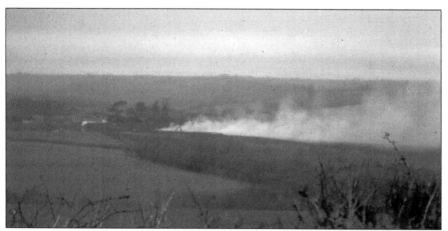

A funeral pyre burning on Dartmoor in Devon during 2001.

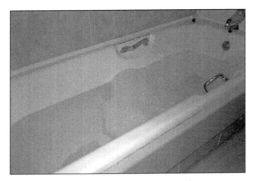

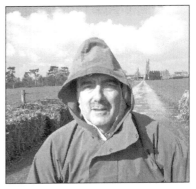

A welcome bath at the end of a day after arriving back from FMD duty in 2001, tired and smelling of disinfectant.

A 'selfie' taken during the 2001 FMD outbreak ready for the long walk up this farm drive.

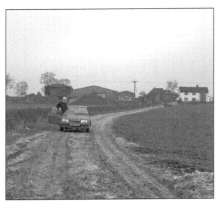

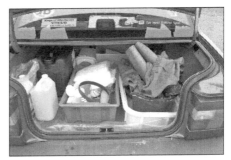

My car stocked with all the essential equipment for FMD visits during 2001.

Waiting at the farm gate for me to undertake my clinical inspection of livestock for evidence of FMD.

A farm under observation for suspect FMD – under Form C restrictions.

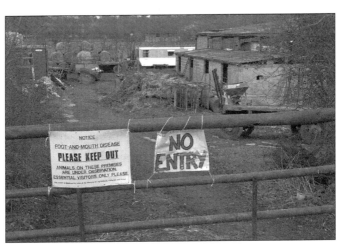

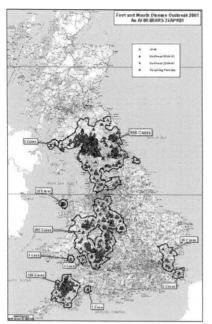

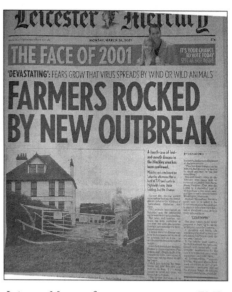

Leicester Mercury front page news: more FMD found in Leicestershire in 2001.

One of the many maps produced during the 2001 FMD epidemic – this was a snapshot view of outbreaks on April 24th 2001.

Chapter 15
Less Disinfectant – and a Move to the Control Teams

I received a phone call from the NDECC and was asked to report to the World Reference Laboratory for Foot-and-Mouth Disease at Pirbright the following day. I packed my case back at the hotel, checked out and drove home. After seven weeks living in hotels, I could at least return home during this particular posting!

I turned up the following day to get my brief and was given 30 days to use my laboratory diagnostic and other skills to set up a national sero-surveillance interface at Pirbright. Basically, the next step after no further clinical disease had been seen in a locality was to prove there was no hidden disease lurking. This could be achieved by bleeding statistically significant numbers of susceptible livestock on each holding within the designated area and testing for evidence of FMD virus activity and specific antibody. Pirbright had the skills and initially the capability to undertake the work but this was a new initiative for the centre and the numbers would be colossal. Also, many of the staff were fully occupied looking at the samples from the outbreak itself. I would be working alongside Pirbright staff, epidemiologists and our own people from the IT department in Weybridge. It was decided early on that this would not be a paper-based exercise but required a separate database.

So it was that by liaising with all concerned we designed a laboratory submission form, methods of collecting blood samples in the field, storing and transporting those samples safely, and receiving and acknowledging their receipt at Pirbright. We also devised methods of increasing testing capability (which quickly meant we had to identify, construct and develop other sites with similar capability at the existing laboratories at Penrith and Luddington), ways to incorporate results from the laboratory into the database and systems for validating and reporting these results. By my 30th day, we had this all in place and it was working well. Sure enough, I received another phone call to be told I was now being moved to a supervisory role running what was referred to as the 'surveillance unit' at the Leeds LDECC. And I was back to staying in hotels again.

When I arrived, the job I was stepping into was not working well and I was asked to try to streamline the way the unit was functioning. Its role was to identify at-risk farms and other livestock units within a 3 km radius of confirmed FMD farms, to serve each one with a Form C restriction notice and to then arrange for a veterinary inspection visit within 24 hours. I was surrounded by maps with different coloured stickers denoting different types of livestock units surrounding the IPs, or infected premises.

It was apparent many of the 'at-risk' farms were not being identified or, if they were, they were not being visited within the agreed timescale. By making a few changes to the system we began to meet the targets expected of us. This was important as we were experiencing a flare-up of infection in the North York Moors area. We had realised we were unaware of many hobby keepers who kept a couple of goats or a couple of sheep, often in a back garden. These were not on our database, yet they remained as susceptible to FMD as those animals kept on a farm and they had to be identified and visited. We arranged for 'patrols' to go out into the urban areas within the restricted zones and ask if anyone knew of friends or neighbours who had sheep or goats in their backyard. We found a few hobby keepers using this method.

This became an important lesson to be learned after the outbreak ceased and legislation was brought in later to ensure anyone owning even one sheep or one goat had to register with Defra, be issued with a holding and herd number and appear on the statutory databases. By the time my three-week period in this team was complete, I was confident we had a reliable system in place and I received a glowing accolade from my line manager at the end of my stint.

Not everything went smoothly, however, and I became a bit of a celebrity over one particular issue. As I've already described, my job was to identify at-risk premises and to send them a Form C notice restricting the movement of susceptible livestock on to or off the premises. The database was never completely accurate and as well as it missing some of the smaller units, I also made contact with some units that had sold their animals and no longer had any susceptible livestock for us to visit. They almost all understood why they had been mistakenly targeted and were happy to accept an apology. All that is except one!

I had contacted a woman to tell her of the serving of a Form C notice on her premises. Unbeknown to me she had no susceptible livestock but she did have a parrot. Her response was to bypass me and contact her local newspaper, which ran a short story quoting my name under a headline 'Has MAFF gone mad?', implying I suspected her parrot had FMD. Unfortunately, *The Sun* national newspaper picked up the story and ran it in a small box under the same heading, again including my name. I never saw it but was told by a colleague that I was actually on page three alongside a scantily clad young woman!

My days were spent in the Leeds office and my nights at a local hotel. This routine continued for the entire three weeks I spent in Yorkshire. I wasn't working such long hours and I at least had the opportunity to use the hotel facilities, such as the health spa and gym. All those working on foot-and-mouth ate every night in the bar area and practically became part of the fixtures and fittings as we sat at the same table most nights. One particular Saturday was memorable. There was a wedding reception taking place in the adjoining function room and we were sitting at our regular table when, to our surprise, the bride in her wedding dress came over to our table. 'We've just found out you are vets working on foot-and-mouth disease and we are farmers and know how hard you've all been working,' she said. This was a pleasant surprise from the criticism we were used to. 'Will you come and join us next door? There is a free bar and buffet and we would be pleased to see you there,' she added. We had a pleasant evening as a result.

After my time in Leeds, I was then sent back to Pirbright to take over the main diagnostic liaison role. I then remained there for the remainder of the outbreak, which was around four months. It was my job to sit between the Pirbright scientists, the veterinary staff in the field and the headquarters staff in London. All calls came through this post, which I shared initially with two other vets, one American and one Australian. As the outbreak diminished I finished up doing the job on my own with relief from AHVLA colleagues on my days off. I had to ensure the paperwork and reference numbers all matched up before releasing results to the NDECC.

I also became increasingly involved in assessing photographs sent in from the field of unusual suspect cases. This was a role I shared with the FMD experts, notably the head of the World Reference Laboratory, Alex Donaldson. When photos were sent in, he and his colleagues asked the simple question: 'Is this FMD or not?' I was then asked to look at them and, ignoring foot-and-mouth, suggest any other possible differential diagnoses. This was a task I did on a day-to-day basis in my real job. We then compared notes to come up with a consensus view to send back to the field investigator who had consulted us.

Towards the culmination of the outbreak, most of my time was being spent not on new incidents but on clearing areas of infection and thus lifting restrictions that had been in place for months on many farms. My last task each day was to receive the blood test serology results as I was responsible for checking each set of farm results to ensure no animal had been incorrectly cleared. If all the results were OK then with one click of my computer mouse that farm was cleared and restrictions could be lifted. I was now returning home with a smile on my face. The end was in sight and I had just brought a smile to another group of farmers, many of whom would have suffered unimaginable heartache and in some cases financial ruin. Perversely perhaps, it was the farms that had disease confirmed and were compensated that suffered less financially than those that were merely closed down for months on end and unable to sell their livestock, but continued having to feed them.

By the end of the outbreak, foot-and-mouth had been confirmed on 2,030 premises across 33 counties in the UK. A total of 3,310,000 sheep, 594,000 cattle, 142,000 pigs and 2,000 other species, such as alpacas and goats, were slaughtered and disposed of, either as a result of confirmed infection or as a precautionary measure. In economic terms, there have been many 'guesstimates' as to the likely cost to UK agriculture. The figure often quoted is around £3 billion with a similar amount lost in tourism revenue as the countryside was effectively shut down during the crisis.

The outbreak handling was criticised severely and with the benefit of hindsight some improvements could have been made. One major difference between this outbreak and the one in 1967 was the massive number of sheep movements that were occurring daily in parallel with the previously reported increase in sheep numbers. These combined to spread infection rapidly around the country, particularly from market dispersals, so we never really caught up with the infection for some time after it was originally identified. To the credit of the effort made by us all we eradicated the Type O pan Asia strain of the disease, a strain that has never to my knowledge been previously eradicated.

I then took over as president of the BCVA and one of my first tasks was to give evidence to a Royal Society enquiry. This culminated in a very thorough and often critical, but thought-provoking report entitled *Foot and Mouth Disease: Lessons to be Learned*. I returned to my full-time post in Winchester at the end of the outbreak hoping that I would never experience FMD in the UK again.

However, in 2007 we received a phone call at the Winchester laboratory from a veterinary practitioner wanting to discuss a problem in a dairy herd that the practice had been consulted over. A number of cows were running high temperatures, were inappetant, and were down in milk yield. Our job as laboratory-based vets was to discuss such cases with our practice colleagues, offering help and advice where we could, and examining any samples that might be taken. There was a nasal discharge and some mouth lesions – and FMD was suggested as a possible differential diagnosis.

This suspicion of FMD was reported to the local animal health office, which immediately despatched a veterinary officer to examine the animals and confirm or rule out FMD. The initial report back to London headquarters was negative, but fortunately the report was made back to the head of the notifiable disease unit, who was immediately concerned about the geographical location of this farm in the village of Normandy in Surrey. The VO was asked to revisit and sample for FMD, and to our surprise the results came back as positive. After only six years, FMD was back.

We immediately knew that the source of the virus had to be either Pirbright or the adjoining pharmaceutical laboratory and vaccine manufacturer; the virus, when typed, was a known laboratory strain of virus carried by both facilities ('01 BFS67-like' FMD virus). We later found out that the virus had escaped from damaged drains to surface water and mud. This, in turn, was picked up by contractor vehicle wheels, which were then parked near the cattle that succumbed to the disease on the farm in Normandy. This gives an excellent indication as to the potential for this devastating virus to spread given the chance.

Disease confirmation was made public on Friday evening and I received a phone call on Saturday morning to report to the Defra headquarters in Page Street in London to help set up the NDECC. I was specifically asked with two colleagues to set up the disease reporting team (DRT), essentially by commandeering desks, telephones, computers and some space. This was a new venture and one that had evolved during the 2001 outbreak. The vets in the DRT were to be the first point of contact from the field to discuss the clinical picture on a one-to-one basis. As a VIO, my skill was in diagnosing problems and specifically looking at differential diagnoses – i.e. what else could the problem potentially be?

I remained in this role as the lead vet throughout the outbreak, aided by colleagues from other laboratories. We took the initial calls, mainly from the LDECC in Guildford as all cases were confined to a very small area around Pirbright. However, the whole country was put under an immediate standstill as a result of recommendations from the Lessons Learned enquiry and it was inevitable we would also be receiving calls about suspected cases from all around the UK. We recorded the location of each new case and allocated it an FMD reference sequential number. The VO on the spot would then be asked to phone their report back to our team, when we would effectively debrief them. I needed to know basic facts such as temperature, whether there were lesions, where they were located if they had lesions, how big they were, how many were present, how many animals were affected and so on. This discussion culminated in a joint assessment as to whether or not we could rule infection out, sample and place under restriction or slaughter immediately on clinical grounds alone. Our team received universal praise from the field as we could effectively help VOs make up their minds by considering other potential causes. Admittedly, we were under far less pressure than our counterparts had been in 2001 so we did have the luxury of time in our favour.

On my second day I took a call from a VO out on a suspect farm who thought he had found FMD in two animals. 'They are salivating and I can see lesions in their mouths', he said. 'Hang on, there is another one, and possibly one more over there'. Cases were developing in front of his eyes. I attracted the attention of a more senior colleague, who immediately called over the chief veterinary officer, both of whom were then reading my notes over my shoulder (and I have pretty awful writing). They immediately gave me the authority to confirm disease and arrangements were put in place to carry out the necessary action.

I had not experienced working at the NDECC in 2001 but I enjoyed (if this is the correct word) the experience in 2007. The decision makers were all around me and we received regular visitors, including the Prime Minister, Gordon Brown, the various Defra ministers and the Defra permanent secretary. The chief veterinary officer and her deputy were on hand, as were the representatives of a wide range of organisations drawn together to control the outbreak. Twice each day we had a 'bird table' meeting, a style of conference brought in by the army in 2001 where everyone involved gathers around a central point, with others on the telephone from around the country, while we were all brought up to date with what was happening in the different sections. It always began with our report detailing the number of report cases and the outcome, with a rolling case tally. This was mainly given by one of the senior vets but I began doing this later in the outbreak.

I also had to provide a situation report at the end of each day to the cabinet office in Downing Street for the emergency Cobra meeting that took place on most days. Cobra stands for cabinet office briefing room and refers to the location for a type of crisis response committee set up to coordinate the actions of bodies within the government in response to crises such as FMD.

What did surprise me in 2007 was the openness Defra had with the media about what was happening each day. I used to phone Gerry as I left Page Street to head home each day and she would say, for example: 'Oh, I see you've put *a well-known public attraction with farm livestock* accessible to the public under restriction'. That was true as we suspected FMD there one day but I had only served the notice that same afternoon and disease was ruled out the following day!

The outbreak was much smaller and more easily managed than 2001 and I settled quickly into a routine of commuting daily to and from London by train from Winchester to Waterloo. I joined the lines of commuters waiting on the platform to catch the 6.30am train and I often didn't get home until gone 9pm.

I also stayed occasionally in a hotel across the road from Page Street where, from some rooms, I could even see my desk.

Many lessons had been learned and applied between these two outbreaks, the most significant of which was a complete standstill being brought in on all livestock movements across the UK. This move successfully confined the outbreak to the south-east of England, with only eight confirmed cases in total. Nevertheless, further hardship was caused to livestock keepers, most of whom had recovered from the problems of six years earlier. Although we received a significant number of 'report cases' of suspicion of disease, these were all ruled out following local inspection by regional veterinary staff. We were concerned that complacency could set in once it became clear that cases were confined to this small area of Surrey and extensive epidemiological modelling was used to create a number of 'what if' scenarios. These were made available to the farming press to ensure everyone kept on their toes and that no illicit animal movements would take place nor the disease be unreported.

As an example, I took a call from an abattoir in north-east England where a vet had expressed concern about lambs with mouth lesions during her inspection and correctly notified the local animal health office. A veterinary officer had gone to investigate and was unable to rule out FMD, hence the call to ourselves on the NDECC. The abattoir was closed immediately, the gates were shut and all staff told they must remain on site while the incident was investigated. Lorries quickly began queuing outside waiting to unload their livestock cargo but the gates remained closed. Not surprisingly, the local media quickly got wind of this and were already reporting as the event unfolded. If this was indeed FMD, then the problem would not be at the abattoir but on the farms of origin.

Luckily, the abattoir driver was still on the premises so his vehicle was contained within the complex and disinfected. It transpired the sheep in this consignment had originated from two separate farms and veterinary officers were sent immediately to each to inspect the live animals remaining for evidence of FMD, which should have been clearly evident if it was there. The drill in such cases is for the veterinary officers who visit the two farms and the vet remaining in the abattoir to discuss the case together and come up with a consensus view. It was this final view that we awaited in London. They were happy to rule out disease as the abattoir lesions were undoubtedly orf and there was widespread evidence of this disease on both premises. The abattoir was eventually reopened during the late afternoon and staff were allowed to leave, although several mothers had already been licensed off to collect their children from school.

The cases all occurred during August and September, although there was a period when it was thought the outbreak south of Pirbright was over only for it to re-emerge a few miles away to the north. Movement restrictions remained in place through the remainder of the autumn, however, until a large scale surveillance exercise testing thousands of blood samples had been completed and no hidden pockets of infection could be found. The country was again granted its FMD-free status by late December.

Unbeknown to me, another notifiable exotic disease known as bluetongue first arrived in the UK during this foot-and-mouth outbreak. We were aware this disease had appeared suddenly in Holland and epidemiological investigations suggested it had originated from sub-Saharan Africa – a big leap! Bluetongue is a midge-transmitted disease that affects a similar species range as FMD. It causes signs that are similar, namely sores and erosions in the mouth and feet, but with other signs including nasal erosions that can be particularly severe over the muzzle of cattle. The name bluetongue was coined to describe the cyanosis that can follow in sheep when a copious amount of fluid builds up in the airways. Affected animals gasp for breath with the tongue going blue as the condition progresses.

We received a call from the Bury St Edmunds office in Suffolk to inform us a veterinary officer was heading out to visit a Highland cow that was showing signs of FMD. Luckily, the VO was experienced and he didn't think the picture was typical but requested that he sample for FMD, place restrictions on the farm as if disease were suspected and await overnight results. This we did and the test results came back negative. It was not FMD but the lesions were severe and there was severe crusting and ulceration of the muzzle. The FMD restrictions were lifted and replaced immediately with similar ones put in place for suspected bluetongue. A fresh set of samples were taken and bluetongue was confirmed.

Disease is dynamic and constantly changing. The emergence of bluetongue into northern Europe and its entry into the UK via a cloud of midges blown across the Channel at a time when we were already dealing with another important disease shows just how important it is to have a robust disease surveillance process in place.

Although exercises simulating outbreaks of notifiable disease were undertaken prior to the 2001 FMD outbreak, they received greater attention and public scrutiny in the years that followed. They are given code names such as Exercise Silver Birch, which was undertaken in 2010 to evaluate the Defra response to a simulated outbreak of FMD, and Exercise Walnut, undertaken in 2013 and involving a suspect outbreak of classical swine fever.

I was asked to take part in Exercise Hawthorn in April 2006. This was a two-day exercise co-ordinated from London surrounding a hypothetical outbreak of highly pathogenic avian influenza, an infection causing global concern at the time as it was causing severe illness and death in people around the world. I travelled to London the evening before the exercise was due to start and was checking into my hotel when a headline that came on the television displaying BBC News 24 in the lobby caught my eye: Avian influenza confirmed in the UK. My first thought was that the BBC was involved in our simulation exercise, but clearly this was real. Just as we were about to start our exercise, we were suddenly faced with the real thing. Hawthorn was immediately aborted but we were then to be tested by reality rather than the often false hypothetical situations we were asked to work through in other simulation exercises.

The UK had already been undertaking an ongoing surveillance exercise, effectively monitoring deaths in wild birds at the regional laboratories, and I had carried out many of these screenings myself. All tests for avian influenza had so far proved negative, but a dead swan found in Cellardyke, a coastal village in Fife in south-west Scotland, in early April 2006 had tested positive for the 'deadly H5N1 strain of bird flu', as the headline I had seen on the hotel television referred to it.

I returned to Winchester the following day as one of the first tasks was to step up the amount of surveillance to assess whether this was a one-off or we were potentially facing a real incursion of the disease. Although Defra was concerned about the potential risk to human health, there was also a real threat of a potentially devastating effect on the UK poultry sector in which mass mortality could seriously hit the nation's food supplies.

Control measures were put in place immediately around Cellardyke, with the establishment of 3 km protection and 10 km surveillance zones. A wild bird risk area of 2,500 sq km was also declared. This meant at the time that:

- Poultry owners within this wild bird risk area had to keep birds indoors or, if this was not possible, ensure they were kept away from wild birds.
- Bird transport within the 10 km surveillance zone would be curbed and gatherings banned.
- Poultry within the 3 km protection zone had to be kept indoors and would be tested.

The wild bird risk zone put in place contained 175 registered poultry premises, with 3.1 million poultry. About 48 of these were free-range premises with 260,000 birds, which were obviously at greater risk of exposure to infected wild birds. This gives the reader an immediate impression of the scale of some of the scenarios that Defra is faced with and often, unfairly in my view, criticised.

Not surprisingly, this incident received full media attention as the world's press seemed to converge on this small Scottish village. It was the first item on the main news bulletins and was the lead headline on the front of the morning newspapers. The general public were understandably concerned and calls began flooding in about dead birds found all around the UK. There was concern these deaths, that occurred every day even in the absence of avian influenza, could be the result of this deadly virus. Defra advice at that time was to contact its local offices and laboratories to arrange for any suspect birds to be collected and examined as part of the ongoing surveillance exercise.

The Winchester catchment area of SE England has a relatively high urban human population, and as a result we were absolutely overwhelmed with dead birds to examine. On the Monday of the week after the isolation had been made in Scotland, the Winchester laboratory where I was based received over 100 yellow polythene bags, each of which contained one or more dead birds for post-mortem examination and sampling. This had to be undertaken alongside our routine work, and we really struggled to keep up with this constant flow.

The work was difficult, particularly as we had to wear full protective gear including an airstream helmet that encased our heads completely and contained a battery supplying a flow of air over our faces. These were hot and uncomfortable during warmer weather. The numbers continued to increase but there was the positive benefit in that the very detailed tissue sampling exercise that we used initially quickly became simplified as key sampling sites and sample types yielding the most consistent results were identified. Nevertheless, we had to work on Saturdays, Sundays and bank holidays to keep up with the constant throughput of birds. It also became apparent that swans were very good sentinels of infection in that they seemed to be very susceptible to the virus, as did some duck breeds and other waterfowl. We began to be more selective and accepted these types of birds whenever we could.

As ever, there were the more amusing incidents, such as the several occasions when members of the public reported 'dead swans' to Defra, which sent out its field staff to collect them only to find a floating white article of clothing in a pond. Three reports were also received about 'dead swans' being clearly visible in a field adjoining a main road in Surrey. On each occasion the field operatives sent to investigate were chased away by these swans, which had found a nice sheltered spot in which to lie in the sun. My own favourite was a call I took from a member of the public who had found two dead blackbirds on the road near where he lived. At the time we were only focusing on swans and other waterfowl but he was very insistent that I must investigate or he would report me to his MP, a threat I have received on more than one occasion for other reasons! Having asked him more about the birds, he was pretty sure they might have been hit by a car but could still be infected with bird flu. In these circumstances it is often easier to comply, which I did. The birds duly arrived the following day. They were indeed blackbirds but had been completely flattened and came to us in an envelope each with the appearance of a pancake! I harvested what tissue I could collect and wasn't in the least bit surprised to receive a final negative avian influenza result.

Monitoring wild bird losses continues today and Defra now has an effective team focusing on wildlife threats to the human population, including continuing surveillance for avian influenza and for another potential threat from West Nile virus.

As I write this account, the number of veterinary laboratories is to be cut drastically as the government spending cuts are enacted through an exercise known as Surveillance 2014.

Can we continue to have the confidence we can recognise these potentially devastating diseases and, more importantly, do we have the skills and resources needed to control them if and when they emerge?

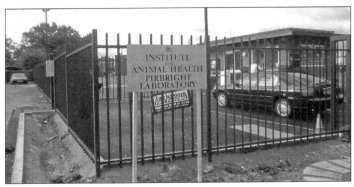

World Reference Laboratory at Pirbright in Surrey where I was based towards the end of the 2001 FMD epidemic.

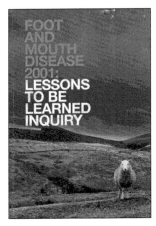

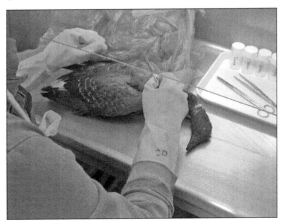

The 'Lessons to be Learned' FMD enquiry report of the handling of the 2001 FMD epidemic.

A goose being examined in a safety cabinet for evidence of highly pathogenic avian influenza infection as part of a national surveillance exercise.

Chapter 16
You've Got to be Kidding!

As a young boy growing up in Church Lench I often saw Amy, who rented the land next to my father's, and her beloved goats. I was always impressed with her knowledge, dedication and obvious love for these fascinating creatures. I could be very imaginative and say that, as I was born under Capricorn, it was perhaps inevitable I would develop an interest in the goat. I was also born in the Chinese year of the ox, so again was it inevitable that I also developed my lifelong interest in cattle? Make of this what you will!

It was while working in Carmarthen that I first became aware of a small and growing enterprise in Pembrokeshire that was encouraging smallholders to move into dairy goat keeping as a local entrepreneur had identified a market selling frozen goat curd to France. This was at the time akin to selling coals to Newcastle – France had a well-developed goat sector, we did not. As the Welsh government of the day was giving out grants and subsidies to set up these enterprises, it also wanted more information and intelligence. It was suggested to me that I make contact with them and essentially become the Welsh goat expert. I immediately joined the Goat Veterinary Society, a small specialist division of the British Veterinary Association, whose members include vets who have an interest in the species, and goat owners.

I had also seen an advertisement in *Farmers Weekly* for a week-long study tour of France, essentially looking at its dairy goat sector. I asked to go on this and was accepted. During this visit, I had the chance to meet a variety of UK goat keepers and talk to them about their animals and how they managed them, alongside a series of visits to French farms. It was an extremely useful experience and really ignited my interest in the species as we were able to see not only the French system of management, but also some of the diseases they were experiencing. At that time, caprine arthritis encephalitis (CAE) and caseous lymphadenitis (CLA) were both serious problems with disease evident on many farms we visited. I had never come across either in the UK. We also visited a small ruminant dairy research unit in Nantes, giving another perspective on the sector.

I returned to Wales full of enthusiasm for the goat, although due to the small number in the UK, I saw very few compared to my heavy cattle and sheep case load in Carmarthen. Following an article I produced for *Farmers Weekly* describing my goat experiences in France, I was asked to speak at the next meeting of the Goat Veterinary Society at the National Agricultural Centre at Stoneleigh in Warwickshire. My subject was metacestode diseases of the goat, a problem we saw very commonly in sheep in Wales. This presented as gid, a parasitic cyst in the brain, or hydatidosis, parasitic cysts in multiple organs such as the liver and lung, although I had never come across the disease in goats and to this day have only encountered it twice. So began a long association with the society and I am currently its chairman. I have now spoken more times than anyone at society meetings and I have written more papers in the journal, which I have also edited for the past seven years.

This interest also came to the attention of the British Goat Society (BGS), a small group of mainly hobby and pedigree keepers based predominantly in the UK. I was asked if I would become one of its honorary veterinary surgeons, to which I consented, and it is a position I still hold. I began speaking to groups of goat owners on a fairly regular basis as their honorary vet and became concerned about the constant criticism of my fellow veterinary colleagues. I was told: 'My vet has no real interest in goats', or, more worryingly: 'My vet knows nothing about goats'. I also heard: 'My vet treats my goat as if it were a cow or a sheep and doesn't seem to realise they are not the same'. I was less worried about the third statement than I was about the first two. There are many similarities in the approach a vet takes to all three as they are all ruminants but there are some often subtle differences.

I approached the BGS committee armed with these comments and concerns and asked if it would consider sponsoring a lecture at one of the UK vet schools to undergraduates. I hoped this would stimulate an interest in goats and increase the knowledge of veterinary undergraduates prior to them qualifying and going into practice. I stated I would be prepared to undertake these if the universities were interested. The committee agreed and I made contact with a colleague I knew through the BCVA at Glasgow University, who agreed to find a slot for me. I produced a set of notes to accompany my lecture, at that time all on slide transparencies. The session ran for around two hours and proved successful. Soon, other colleges wanted to follow this initiative. In time, I was visiting London (my old college), Bristol, Liverpool, Glasgow and Edinburgh each year and Cambridge on an occasional basis. I was also invited to give some introductory lectures on goats in the first year at the newly created University of Nottingham School of Veterinary Medicine and Science. I have continued to undertake this visit annually to four vet schools, with occasional visits to the others depending on curricular demand. After nearly 20 years, I must have spoken to somewhere between 4,000 and 7,000 undergraduates, the majority of whom are now in practice in the UK. Hopefully they are able to prove to goat owners that they have not only an interest in this fascinating species but also have some ideas on how best to manage their health and welfare. It is one change I hope I've had some influence over!

The goat sector in the UK is small, with around 98,000 animals in total compared to 10 million cattle and around 30 million sheep. Nevertheless, it is a very diverse sector. The hobby and pedigree sector supported by the British Goat Society has changed very little but in contrast we have seen a dramatic change in the commercial dairy goat sector. The frozen curd enterprise in Wales never really took off but in its place we saw increasingly larger units set up producing liquid milk for the UK retail market. This sector makes up around 33 per cent of our total goat population, with individual units having up to 4,500 milking females.

In turn, I have learned an immense amount about goat behaviour from the owners I have met during my time as honorary vet. Goats are incredibly intelligent animals and owners can develop quite remarkable bonds with them as a result. These connections can be so strong that some goats will pine to the point of being ill if their owner goes away on holiday for even a few days. They are great escapologists, seemingly able to squeeze through the tiniest of gaps, and are always trying to reach something more interesting to eat than you have given them. They investigate everything with their mouths and this, coupled with their ability to reach up to 2 metres, means many can open gate catches and escape or chew through electric cables and electrocute themselves. One skill a goat owner has to learn quickly is how to make a goat pen, paddock or building goat-proof, as opposed to merely making it livestock-proof.

An observation I have repeated to students many times came from a stockman who, before he built up and ran his own commercial dairy goat herd, worked on a dairy cow unit milking cows. 'The difference between milking cows and milking goats is that you have to push cows into the parlour to milk them, whereas you push goats out in the opposite direction'. This observation is highly relevant. They are inquisitive, get bored easily and enjoy anything happening around them – and the milking routine is just another game to them. Once the milking machine starts up on the commercial units, goats gather around the gates waiting to be first out. Some can open the gates and let themselves out. They rush to be first into the parlour and many will then try to get back in again after they have been milked.

There has been a strong and very welcome move during my lifetime as a vet to ensure that farm animals kept intensively or semi-intensively have a 'happy life', and much of this is down to improved environmental enrichment. A single bale of straw placed in a paddock or pen can provide hours of fun and large empty plastic drums can be climbed into, balanced on top of or even used for hiding inside. One Angora herd I visited had chairs placed around the pens and the goats jumped up and sat on them as if they were in my waiting room!

Goats genuinely enjoy the company of humans and make excellent animals to keep in pet corners at zoos and other animal collections. I have never encountered an aggressive goat – an excessively playful and inquisitive goat yes – but never aggressive. This inquisitiveness and love of human attention often makes it problematic to examine them when other goats are around. You can be examining one goat with your stethoscope while another chews your sleeve and others steal equipment you have brought in with you. I took my eldest daughter Maddy with me to a goat unit when she was about six and at a time when she wanted to be a vet like her dad. Armed with her junior doctor's case, she came into the pen with me to watch me examining some lame goats. I became engrossed in the task until I heard a rather plaintive, 'Dad, Dad, Dad', getting ever louder and slightly more anxious each time. I looked around and all I could see was the junior doctor's case being held as high above Maddy's head as she could manage, but I could not see her. She was completely surrounded by goats, all stretching their heads up to get at the mysterious case she was holding.

Having spoken to so many veterinary undergraduates during my visits to the UK vet schools to talk about goats, each of whom gets a copy of my goat notes, it is hardly surprising that I receive phone calls and emails on a very regular basis asking for help and advice. Many of the photos I use for these lectures have been sent to me by people looking for a clinical opinion. Calls are many and varied but may be to ask for help with a skin problem, worms, vaccination programmes and a wide variety of other problems and conditions. I help wherever I can, sometimes referring them on to other colleagues specialising in surgery, which has never been my forte.

I also get a number of enquiries from goat owners and sadly they still often comment on their vet's lack of knowledge or interest in goats, making it very difficult for me to get too involved as I never wish to be appearing to undermine a colleague. My approach in such a situation has always been to get the owner's vet to contact me directly and this often works.

The BGS has a discussion forum, which is a Yahoo member-only group. This is an extremely useful medium through which to exchange problems, solutions and a variety of other topics of goat interest. I tend to step in when there are direct requests for veterinary advice or occasionally when I think that discussions are giving misleading or incorrect advice.

I have also been invited to speak about the UK goat sector and its health and welfare problems at conferences in Denmark and Norway. These are always useful visits and many valuable contacts are made. They can also be extremely thought-provoking, particularly when during my trip to Denmark I was discussing how we disbud goat kids in the UK and some of the problems we encounter with both the procedure and its implications. I could sense my audience was not with me and quickly found out the procedure is banned in that country.

For the uninitiated, the majority of goats will eventually grow horns and, for a variety of reasons I'll explain, we destroy the germinative bud of the developing horn by thermocautery under either local or general anaesthetic. It is more or less a routine procedure on both large and small goat holdings in this country, aimed at preventing problems related to the horns injuring other goats, goat keepers or others in the vicinity. The procedure also prevents goats getting caught up in fencing or hedgerows. I described these reasons to my Danish audience, all of whom said none posed a problem for them and they kept goats together in large groups or small groups with very few if any horn-related incidents. I returned to the UK armed with this information and resolved to change things over here. However, despite me describing the Danish experience, I have singularly failed to change the mindset of goat owners in the UK. Perhaps I should be more vociferous!

In 2014 as I complete this book, the UK goat sector is bracing itself for what could be a developing problem related to bovine TB. We saw no TB in goats from the early 1950s until 2007, but since then we have had two small incidents on smallholdings in Wales and Wiltshire. There was one further incident involving Golden Guernseys on a number of linked goat units, each of which purchased animals incubating disease from a unit in Wales with unrecognised or undisclosed infection. The index cases were all considered to be straightforward spillovers of infection from the local wildlife population (predominantly badgers) as each incident developed in known TB hotspots and involved the local geographical strain, or spoligotype, of bovine TB. Similar problems have also been identified in alpacas and in sheep – again apparently associated with spillover of infection and subsequent spread within infected herds.

The vast majority of our larger commercial goat herds are housed all year for the control of worms, to which goats have very poor resistance. They remain susceptible throughout their lives and are denied grazing out in fields and paddocks. As a result, it has been assumed that they would be unlikely to develop TB, being effectively protected within their buildings. However, two commercial herds are currently under restriction as TB has been confirmed. The milk leaving these farms is perfectly safe for human consumption as it is pasteurised. The significant and financially damaging problem the goat sector currently faces though is that goats are not included under UK TB legislation. Hence, no compensation is payable to assist such farm owners to rid themselves of TB, unlike the legislation and compensation paid to cattle farmers. It is anticipated that goats will eventually be brought into existing legislation as consultation is proposed.

Just as this TB incident was getting into the public domain, Gerry received a phone call from someone at the BBC Radio 4 *Farming Today* programme asking to speak to me. 'He's on the golf course', was her reply, as I had just taken up the game. Gerry took a message and I phoned back, whereupon I was asked to take part in a radio interview to be broadcast the following morning, which could be recorded that day. I agreed to go the Radio Solent studio in Winchester for a link-up with the London studio. I was somewhat taken aback when I arrived to be told it was a locked room for which the doorman of the building had a key. He let me in and, sure enough, I was totally on my own with a crib sheet to tell me which buttons to press and what dials to turn. This did add to the tension somewhat. A phone rang and, with my headphones in place and the microscope switched on, I eventually did the interview, giving my views on the outbreak and some background information about the goat sector in the UK. It wasn't until the broadcast the following day that I realised I had been effectively responding on behalf of the UK goat sector to the previous item, an interview with Owen Paterson, then the secretary of state at Defra!

The amount of data we had on goats in the UK was minimal when I first became interested, particularly in relation to the use of medicines, very few of which have marketing authorisations for use in the animal. Through the work of the GVS – and hopefully I have played my part – I am now intensely proud of where we are today compared to 20 years ago. Goats in the UK have benefited and I am confident their health and welfare has improved as a result of our work.

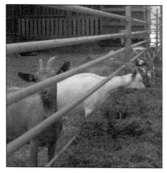

Goats in Denmark kept intensively with horns; why don't we follow their example in the UK!

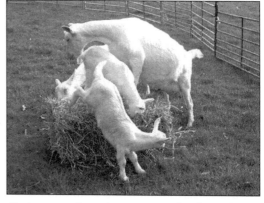

Environmental enrichment – great fun from a bale of straw.

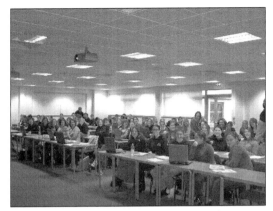

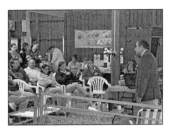

Me talking to British Goat Society members at the Royal Show held at the National Agricultural Centre in Warwickshire.

Undergraduate students at the new Nottingham School of Veterinary Medicine and Science during one of my half-day sessions on goat health and welfare.

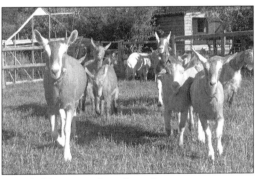

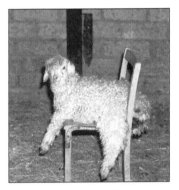

Pet / hobby goats – friendly and gregarious.

An Angora goat on a chair waiting for me – there were several placed around a pen for environmental enrichment.

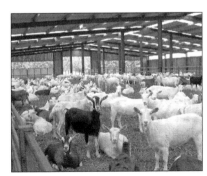

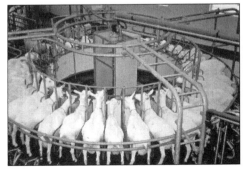

A UK commercial dairy goat unit, a developing sector.

A rotary carousel milking parlour on a UK commercial dairy goat farm.

Chapter 17
Some Final Thoughts

I retired from my full-time career in the AHVLA in May 2013 and have been undertaking some consultancy work ever since, having been loath to give up completely and head for the golf course. One area I have been involved in is setting up a completely new veterinary school at the University of Surrey. Through contacts with former colleagues at AHVLA, I was invited in on a number of days to work up a curriculum for the university to put before the Royal College of Veterinary Surgeons to gain its support for the course. This was a new, but highly challenging exercise that I have enjoyed. The curriculum is so innovative in many areas that I genuinely wish I could enrol and start my veterinary studies all over again! Somewhat ironically, it completes the loop of my veterinary career as I started and am finishing at a veterinary college. I have also been helping set up a field post-mortem site with WestPoint, a neighbouring veterinary practice, and have been involved in providing some training in post-mortem techniques to groups of young intern vets in the practice. I have recently been appointed a visiting reader in the Faculty of Health and Medical Sciences, at the University of Surrey.

The activities which I have been engaged in during my time working in the state veterinary service have included dealing with notifiable / exotic diseases such as FMD, BSE, Bluetongue and Avian Influenza; completing ongoing daily work to identify, categorise and control new and emerging diseases; and identifying potential food safety concerns. Underpinning these activities is a need to have a robust animal health surveillance programme in place. During this same time period, the number of laboratories has gradually reduced.

Shortly before I retired, I was asked to join a high-profile team to develop a surveillance programme for the future – driven predominantly by the need to reduce the Defra budget in line with all other government departments at that time. The group was chaired by Professor Dirk Pfeiffer, Professor of Veterinary Epidemiology at the Royal Veterinary College, and included a number of representatives from veterinary, farming and government circles. It was referred to as 'Surveillance 2014', and met for the first time in January 2012, with a remit to produce its final report by March 2012.

We were charged at that time with developing an increased surveillance strategy for England and Wales, whilst at the same time facing the financial constraints placed on all government departments. Increasing the number of veterinary laboratories was never an option, and we somehow had to improve what we had, with an inevitable reduction in both government laboratories and government veterinary and laboratory staff. We were provided with a series of options for rationalisation (effectively laboratory closures) based on livestock population densities, particularly considering the main livestock species in each area. The report referred to as the 'Surveillance Advisory Group Final Report' (March 2012) came up with a series of options regarding laboratory closures and enhancement of remaining laboratories. Greater use was to be made of private veterinary practitioners, who had always been our 'eyes and ears', being on farms more regularly than we were, and knowing their clients' livestock systems. The 'vision' was that private vets (many of whom already undertake work on behalf of government, such as TB-testing cattle through designated roles as 'official veterinarians' or 'OV') would be trained in undertaking more post-mortem examinations themselves (so-called field post mortem examinations). This increased number of post-mortems would be available to Defra as part of the programme to supplement the increased size and capacity of the remaining laboratories. A transport infrastructure would also be put in place to enable carcass collection from farms and onward delivery to a designated laboratory if potential new and emerging diseases were suspected or if serious outbreaks of disease required more specialised investigation.

This enhancement was inevitable, and as a member of the group, I supported what we had recommended. The problem, however, was implementation; sadly, two years after the event, many laboratories have closed, and many of the veterinary practitioners who were served by these laboratories have been suddenly left with no easy local access to post-mortem facilities for their clients. More importantly, in this new era, they have been left with no training in how to undertake 'better post-mortem examinations'. My local laboratory at Winchester was forced to close ahead of schedule at the end of May 2014, suddenly leaving SE England with no local laboratory – and again no training had been put in place. The letter sent out to each practice described the main option open to them – namely using the nearest laboratory at Bury St Edmunds in East Anglia, over 140 miles away, and also the surveillance centre at the Royal Veterinary College. Currently, arrangements are in place for carcasses to be transported to these laboratories at no cost to those making the submission subject to certain criteria.

I repeat my earlier statement. Do we have the confidence that we can recognise incursions of exotic disease into the UK and have the skills and resources to control them if they emerge? Equally, have we the ongoing daily surveillance needed to identify potentially important new and emerging diseases and potential food chain threats? In a nutshell, I was always working under the guise of ensuring that we could recognise the 'next BSE' if ever such a problem occurred again and this must still be an ongoing priority no matter how the Surveillance 2014 rationalisation programme is eventually implemented.

I had the opportunity to give something back to my profession in 2002 when I agreed in the early hours of the morning in a central Birmingham penthouse hotel suite (and after a surplus of alcohol) to join a cycle ride from London to Edinburgh. I was at that time president of the BCVA and was at the British Small Animal Veterinary Association congress as the guest of its president, and in the company of presidents of the other major veterinary organisations and our wives. It was the idea of Stephen Ware, at that time president of the Royal College of Veterinary Surgeons.

Stephen's idea was that when we had each completed our presidential years, we would join forces relay fashion to cycle from British Veterinary Association headquarters in London to the BVA congress to be held in Edinburgh. It was to be known as the Tour de Vets, our take on the Tour de France, but much lower key. In a drunken haze we all agreed and all promptly forgot about it, except Stephen who made contact with us some time later. In his view, it was to be our way of giving back something to our profession. I was to ride the last four legs of around 70 miles each day through Yorkshire, Cumbria and into Scotland and on to Edinburgh, which I did.

We each had a chosen charity and mine was Send a Cow, an extremely worthwhile overseas charity I would urge every reader to consider supporting. Its work provides poor families with the skills they need to build new lives free from poverty and hunger by providing training, livestock, seeds and support; it restores hope and creates stronger communities. For every one person the charity helps, ten more go on to benefit.

Central to its work is its 'pass it on' principle. Families working with Send a Cow pass on young livestock, seeds or training to others, and so on. This not only builds stronger communities, it allows the charity to help even more people to develop skills, confidence and self-respect. I raised around £2,000 due partly to the humbling generosity of my family but in particular to many members of the veterinary profession. Some of these were well known to me, but many were total strangers with a common bond of having an MRCVS (member of the Royal College of Veterinary Surgeons) after our name.

I was an elected trustee of the Animal Welfare Foundation from 2008 for two successive three-year terms, elected at the same time as Emma Milne, one of the original vets featured on the TV documentary programme *Vets in Practice*. AWF is a UK-based charity that I would again urge readers to consider supporting. This charity is the veterinary profession's own animal welfare charity and is run by a group of trustees, all of whom are veterinary surgeons concerned about a wide range of animal welfare issues and sharing a collective vision of all animals living healthy and contented lives free from pain and suffering. Its mission statement is:

'To improve the welfare of all animals through veterinary science, education and debate'.

There have been a number of generous legacies and donations over the 30 years the charity has been in existence and this has enabled the funding of some excellent animal welfare associated projects that have been predominantly undertaken by researchers at UK veterinary schools. Once each year the charity holds a discussion forum in central London, during which specific welfare-related topics are debated by the audience. This event culminates with a reception at the House of Commons, during which we have the opportunity to lobby invited MPs over a range of issues. The charity has also funded animal welfare lectureships at Bristol, Glasgow and Liverpool veterinary schools.

It has been a cathartic experience conveying one's life to paper – everyone should try it! I worked through some difficult times, most notably the terrible FMD outbreak of 2001 and a further incursion in 2007, and also witnessed at first hand the BSE epidemic almost from day one to its conclusion.

Despite these often harrowing times, I can still admit to having thoroughly enjoyed my working life as a veterinary surgeon, something that I accept that we cannot all say about our choice of career. I can honestly say I have never once woken up and thought 'here we go again, another day on the treadmill'. I have been lucky that very few of my days have ended up as a routine! Certainly there were times in practice when, tucked up in a warm bed, I didn't relish the thought of heading off to some cold building to calve a cow. However, the delivery of a calf with a healthy dam was always just reward for this.

Towards the end of my full-time working career I did gradually become more and more frustrated by the bureaucratic influences – mainly due to health and safety measures – that began to have an impact on my work as a government vet, but I had to accept that it was happening in most working environments.

I have also been very fortunate to have had a series of role models throughout my career, although most of them I suspect may not have known the high regard in which I held each of them. I thank them all and hope I have lived up to the examples they set.

I had a loving and caring family during my childhood and was fortunate to have grown up in a small isolated village, both of these factors giving me an uncomplicated and solid foundation on which to build. It was my grandfather, of course, who set me off on the path to becoming a vet, a career choice I have never for one moment doubted.

Diane gave me the support I needed to fulfil my ambition to become a vet and helped me get on to the ladder that I continued to climb from day one. She also gave me my two lovely daughters, Maddy and Jessica.

It has been my second wife Gerry, however, who has given me her full and total support and the confidence to branch out into areas I never considered within my reach. I achieved the presidency of the BCVA, I am currently chairman of the GVS and have been chairman or president of other British Veterinary Association divisions and local veterinary clinical clubs. I am now a visiting reader at the new University of Surrey School of Veterinary Medicine and am also a visiting lecturer at the London, Liverpool, Bristol and Glasgow vet schools. I have also written a book titled *Goat Health and Welfare: A Veterinary Guide.*

This has been the story of a young boy who aspired to be a veterinary surgeon, eventually achieving his ambition and perhaps far more.

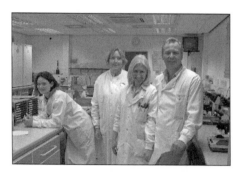

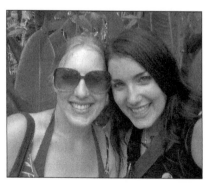

My laboratory technical colleagues were an invaluable part of the regional laboratory team.

My daughters Maddy and Jess.

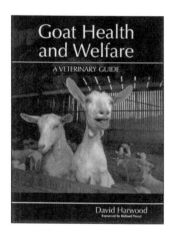

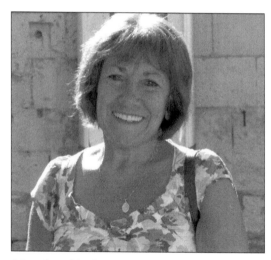

My book 'Goat Health and Welfare' has sold over 3500 copies worldwide.

My wife and 'soulmate' Gerry.